CLINICAL MANUAL

for

ESSENTIALS OF MATERNITY NURSING: FAMILY-CENTERED CARE by

Leonide L. Martin, RN, MS, Dr PH

Sharon J. Reeder, RN, PhD, FAAN

Prepared by

CRACOM Corporation

J. B. Lippincott Company   PHILADELPHIA

NEW YORK   •   ST. LOUIS   •   LONDON

SYDNEY   •   TOKYO

Library of Congress Cataloging-in-Publication Data

Martin, Leonide L.
    Clinical manual for essentials of maternity nursing/Leonide L.
Martin, Sharon J. Reeder.
        p.   cm.
    Includes index.
    ISBN 0-397-54897-4
    1.   Obstetrical nursing.   2.   Nursing assessment.   I.   Reeder,
Sharon J.   II.   Title.
    [DNLM: 1.   Nursing Assessment—handbooks.   2.   Obstetrical
Nursing—handbooks.   WY 39 M381c]
RG951.M3123   1991
610.73′678—dc20
DNLM/DLC
for Library of Congress   90-13645
                                                                    CIP

The authors and publishers have exerted every effort to ensure that
drug selection and dosage set forth in this text are in accord with
current recommendations and practice at the time of publication.
However, in view of ongoing research, changes in government
regulations, and the constant flow of information relating to drug
therapy and drug reactions, the reader is urged to check the package
insert for each drug for any change in indications and dosage and for
added warnings and precautions. This is particularly important when
the recommended agent is a new or infrequently employed drug.

CONTENTS

6   Second Stage of Labor   84

7   Operative Obstetrics   94

8   Third and Fourth Stages of Labor   110

15   Intrapartum Complications   249

16   Postpartum Complications   259

PREFACE

The Clinical Manual for *Essentials of Maternity Nursing* is a useful tool for maternity nursing students or graduate nurses who have chosen maternity nursing as their specialty. The organization of the Clinical Manual provides a quick reference when the nurse's assessment focuses on a special treatment area. The guide is divided into six units that cover normal pregnancy and maternal and newborn care, as well as complications. Each chapter contains pertinent assessment information and where applicable, laboratory values, client self-care education, guides, nursing procedures, and nursing care plans. In addition, drug guides are included that contain information on the drugs most commonly used in pregnancy, labor, delivery, and the neonatal periods. The pocket size makes it easy for nurses to keep pertinent information at their fingertips and helps them provide safe, effective nursing care for maternity clients and their families.

NORMAL PREGNANCY

Chapter 1

MATERNAL NURSING CARE IN THE ANTEPARTUM PERIOD

Optimum antepartal care begins with the thorough collection of data about the client's history, physical status and psychosocial background during the first prenatal visit. Follow-up care at regularly scheduled intervals throughout pregnancy allows opportunity to monitor maternal and fetal status, institute necessary treatment and additional diagnostic tests, and offer ongoing maternal and family support and education.

COMPONENTS OF THE PRENATAL PHYSICAL EXAMINATION

Part examined / Examination technique	Usual findings during pregnancy	Abnormal findings
HEAD AND NECK		
Palpation, inspection with otoscope or ophthalmoscope, and visual inspection of the mouth	Hyperemia of nasal and buccal mucous membranes, slight diffuse enlargement of thyroid (these changes are associated with pregnancy)	Enlarged lymph nodes, thyroid nodules or irregular enlargement, lesions of eyes or mouth, caries and abcesses of teeth, ear infections
CHEST AND HEART		
Auscultation with stethoscope, percussion, and visual inspection	Lungs clear, heart in regular rhythm (occasionally a soft, short functional murmur caused by hemodynamic changes of pregnancy)	Rales, wheezes, rhonchi, irregular cardiac rhythm, nonphysiologic murmurs
BREASTS		
Palpation and visual inspection	Enlargement of breasts, with increased vascular patterns, darkened	Masses of nodules, bloody or serosanguineous nipple discharge, nipple

2

COMPONENTS OF THE PRENATAL PHYSICAL EXAMINATION—continued

Part examined / Examination technique	Usual findings during pregnancy	Abnormal findings
BREASTS—cont'd		
	aerolae with prominent tubercles, colostrum from nipples in later pregnancy; note if nipples are inverted so preparation can be initiated if mother wishes to breast-feed	lesions, erythema, absence of changes associated with pregnancy
SKIN		
Visual inspection	Pigmentation changes (linea nigra, chloasma), enlargement of nevi, appearance of spider angiomas, mottled erythema of hands	Pallor, jaundice, rash, skin lesions
EXTREMITIES		
Visual inspection and palpation, percussion with reflex hammer	Mild pretibial and ankle edema in third trimester, slight edema of hands in hot weather	Limitations of motion; varicosities; more than slight pretibial, hand, or ankle edema; edema of face or sacrum; hyperflexia and clonus

Continued

COMPONENTS OF THE PRENATAL PHYSICAL EXAMINATION— continued

Part examined Examination technique	Usual findings during pregnancy	Abnormal findings
ABDOMEN		
Palpation, visual inspection, auscultation, percussion	Enlarged uterus, palpation of fetal outline in later pregnancy, fetal heart sounds, contractions in last trimester	Uterus too large or too small for dates, absence of fetal heart sounds beyond 10 weeks (using Doppler), transverse lie of fetus, fetal head in fundus, tonic uterine contractions, enlarged liver or spleen
PELVIS		
Speculum examination, bimanual examination with inspection and palpation, collection of specimens	*Speculum examination:* Bluish discoloration of mucosa of vagina and cervix (Chadwick's sign), congested cervix, ectropion cervix in multigravidas, increased leukorrhea *Bimanual examination:* Soft cervix (Goodell's sign), admits a finger or two (depending on gravida and length of pregnancy); softening of lower uterine segment (Hegar's sign); enlarged uterus; fetal head or parts may be felt in lower	*Speculum examination:* Yellow, purulent, frothy, cheesy, white or homogeneous gray, foul-smelling discharge; friable, bleeding lesions of cervix; vaginal lesions; bleeding from cervical os; amniotic fluid loss *Bimanual examination:* Cervix dilated and effaced (unless labor has begun); cervical or vaginal masses; excessive amniotic fluid (uterus unusually enlarged); adnexal masses or fullness; rectal masses;

COMPONENTS OF THE PRENATAL PHYSICAL EXAMINATION—
continued

Part examined Examination technique	Usual findings during pregnancy	Abnormal findings
PELVIS—cont'd		
	uterine segment; gynecoid pelvic configuration *Papanicolaou smear:* Squamous cell metaplasia; negative or normal, adequate or increased estrogen; endocervical cells; hyperplasia that is considered borderline	hemorrhoids; contractions of the pelvic inlet, midpelvis, or outlet *Papanicolaou smear:* Inflammation; presence of *Trichomonas vaginalis* or fungi; diminished or absent estrogen; atypical or suspicious cells; atypical hyperplasia, dysplasia, neoplasia, or carcinoma

LABORATORY TESTS DURING PREGNANCY

Test	Purpose
URINE TESTS	
Urinalysis	
Sugar	Screens for diabetes; evaluated at each visit
Albumin (microscopic)	Screens for preeclampsia; evaluates for kidney stress or renal problems; done at each visit
Urine culture	Diagnoses urinary tract infection; often done routinely on all pregnant women
BLOOD TESTS	
Blood urea nitrogen (BUN), creatinine, total protein, electrolytes	Evaluates renal function and diagnoses renal disease

Continued

LABORATORY TESTS DURING PREGNANCY—continued

Test	Purpose
BLOOD TESTS—cont'd	
Complete blood count (CBC)	
Hematocrit and hemoglobin	Screens for anemia, iron deficiency, folic acid deficiency
White blood cell count	Identifies infectious processes
Differential	Screens for blood disorders and inflammatory conditions
Platelets	Assesses blood clotting mechanism
Hemoglobin electrophoresis	Diagnoses hemoglobinopathies (e.g., sickle cell anemia, thalassemias)
Rh factor and blood type	Alerts care provider to possible incompatibility disease in fetus; identifies blood type in case of hemorrhage
Rh titers	Done when woman is Rh negative and man is Rh positive to assess danger to fetus (rising titer)
Maternal serum α-fetoprotein test (AFP)	Screens for fetal neural tube defects such as anencephaly and myelomeningocele; may also indicate abortion, multiple pregnancy, fetal demise
Rubella antibodies	Determines if woman has developed rubella antibodies
Serologic test for syphilis	Screens for syphilis (if positive, must confirm with fluorescent treponemal antibody absorption [FTA-ABS] test)
Hepatitis viral studies	Screens for hepatitis B antigens and antibodies
Enzyme-linked immunosorbent assay (ELISA)	Screens for human immunodeficiency virus (HIV) in consenting high-risk clients; if positive, must confirm with Western blot test immunofluorescent antibody assay (IFA)
OTHER	
Gonorrhea culture of cervical discharge	Diagnoses gonorrhea; often done routinely because gonorrhea is frequently asymptomatic in women

LABORATORY TESTS DURING PREGNANCY—continued

Test	Purpose
OTHER—cont'd	
Chlamydia smears of cervical discharge	Diagnoses *Chlamydia trachomatis;* often done routinely because *Chlamydia* infections are frequently asymptomatic
Papanicolaou smear of cervical epithelium	Screens for cervical intraepithelial neoplasia, herpes simplex type 2
Tuberculin skin test	Screens high-risk women for tuberculosis
Electrocardiogram (ECG), chest roentgenogram	Evaluates cardiac and pulmonary function (performed when indicated by acute or chronic diseases)

SCHEDULE OF RETURN PRENATAL VISITS

First through sixth month—one visit per month
Seventh through eighth month—one visit every 2 weeks
Ninth month until delivery—one visit per week

Assessments Included in Visits

Each visit
Weight
Blood pressure
Fundal height (McDonald's technique)
Check for edema
Urinalysis for glucose and albumin
Inquiry about symptoms, signs, or problems
Nutrition and appetite
Family and personal problems and adjustment
Prenatal education

10th-12th week and every week thereafter
Fetal heart rate with Doppler ultrasound

20th week and every week thereafter
Fetal heart rate with fetoscope

32-34 weeks
Hematocrit and hemoglobin (more often if anemic)

Middle of ninth month
Pelvic examination (then weekly as indicated)

Others
Rh titers for Rh-negative client with Rh-positive father of baby—
if initially negative, twice more during pregnancy; if positive,
more often as indicated by titer levels
Urine culture as indicated by symptoms or signs
Other examinations and tests as indicated by symptoms or signs

ASSESSMENT

CLIENT ASSESSMENT AND HISTORY

Current pregnancy data
First day of last menstrual period (LMP)
Client's response and adaptation to her pregnancy
Any symptoms experienced since the LMP such as nausea, vom-
iting, urinary frequency, and breast changes
Any vaginal spotting or bleeding, with or without cramping, that
has occurred since the LMP

Past obstetric data
Year of each previous pregnancy
Outcome of each pregnancy (abortion, preterm, fullterm, living, or
stillborn)
Any complications experienced during the antepartum, intrapar-
tum, or postpartum period
Length of labor
Type of delivery (vaginal or cesarean)
Health status of the neonate
Weight of the neonate

Current medical history data
Client's perception of her current health status
Height, weight, and vital signs
Blood type and Rh factor if known
Current use of any licit or illicit substances, including, but not
limited to, alcohol, tobacco, cocaine, heroin, over-the-counter
medications, and prescription drugs
Current acute or chronic disease conditions being treated or mon-
itored by a primary care practitioner

Any known allergies

Eating patterns (a review of client's food intake for the 3 preceding days facilitates nutritional assessment)

Exercise routines

Exposure to communicable diseases since the beginning of pregnancy (especially rubella if not immune)

Illnesses such as colds or influenza since the beginning of pregnancy

Exposure to any teratogenic agent since the beginning of pregnancy

Past medical history data

Childhood diseases

Date of immunizations, particularly rubella

Menstrual history, including age at menarche and description of typical cycle

Date of onset and treatment of diseases such as anemia, asthma, blood dyscrasias, cancer, cardiac disease, diabetes mellitus, endocrinopathy, hypertension, psychiatric disorders, renal or urinary tract diseases, and tuberculosis

Date of occurrence and treatment for sexually transmitted diseases

Dates and types of surgery

Dates and reasons for previous hospitalizations

Dates and number of blood transfusions

Injuries, especially to pelvic structure and organs

Contraceptive history and practice

Sexual practices

Personal characteristics

Age

Racial and ethnic background

Education

Occupation

Support networks, including father of baby, children, other family members, and close friends

Data about father of baby

Age

Height and weight

Racial and ethnic origin

Education

Occupation

Potential health hazards
Current health status
Significant medical history
Any known conditions that are generally transmitted (self or family)
Use of licit or illicit substances, including, but not limited to, alcohol, tobacco, cocaine, heroin, over-the-counter medications, and prescription drugs
Blood type and Rh factor
Response to pregnancy

Family history data
Health status of parents and siblings (if decreased, note cause of death)
Occurrence or history of the following diseases in parents, siblings, and close relatives: cancer, cardiopulmonary diseases, complications of pregnancy, congenital anomalies, diabetes mellitus, hypertension, psychiatric disorders, renal disease, tuberculosis, and vascular disease

IDENTIFICATION OF HIGH-RISK PREGNANCY

Sociodemographic factors
Age
    16 years of age or less
    35 years of age or more
Low socioeconomic status

Factors arising from deviations in health
Obstetric and fetal or neonatal factors
    Parity of 5 or more
    History of spontaneous abortions
    History of ectopic pregnancy
    History of preterm births
    Less than 1 year since previous birth
    History of fetal macrosomia
    History of low birth weight infants
    Contracted pelvis
    Anomalies of the reproductive system
    History of operative deliveries
    History of prolonged true labor
    History of breech deliveries
    History of one or more infants with birth defects

Rh incompatibility or blood group (ABO) sensitization
Currently experiencing multiple pregnancy
Uterine or ovarian tumors
Preexisting medical disorders
  Diabetes mellitus
  Cardiac disease
  Chronic hypertension
  Hemoglobinopathies and other blood dyscrasias
  Hyperthyroidism or hypothyroidism
  Chronic renal disease
  Sexually transmitted diseases
  Malnutrition
  Respiratory disorders such as tuberculosis and emphysema
  Substance abuse, including tobacco
Disorders occurring during pregnancy
  Pregnancy-induced hypertension: preeclampsia and eclampsia
  Gestational diabetes
  Acute infectious diseases
  Sexually transmitted diseases
  Substance abuse, including tobacco
  Hemorrhagic disorders, including placenta previa and abruptio
    placentae
  Hydatidiform mole
  Pyelonephritis
  Multiple pregnancy

CULTURAL CONSIDERATIONS*

Questions involving belief systems surrounding childbearing

Antepartum
Who may have a child?
At what age?
By whom may one have a child?
How many children can one have?
Can one space pregnancies?
What should be the behavior during pregnancy?

---

*Adapted from Griffith S: Childbearing and the concept of culture. JOGN 11(3):181, 1982.

Are there restrictions on the father?
Are there any restrictions on sexual activity?
Who may see and touch certain body parts?
How is a fetus formed?
What are the beliefs about conception?

Intrapartum
What causes labor?
How does one behave during labor?
How should one respond to pain?
Should one take medication?
Where should labor take place?

Postpartum
What general behavior is expected?
What behavior is expected of the father and others?
Are there restrictions on food or activity?

Care of the newborn
When is he or she recognized?
What are the rules for his or her care?
Who cares for the newborn?

ASSESSMENT OF PSYCHOSOCIAL ASPECTS OF PREGNANCY

Family composition
1. Who are the family members (include the extended family)?
    a. What are their ages? What are their relationships to one another?
    b. Where do they live? Do they interact frequently?
    c. Are they "close" emotionally if not physically?
    d. What is the family's relationship to the larger educational community? Is the family involved in community affairs and religious activities? What is its community support structure?

Family functioning
1. How are the roles allocated and differentiated?
    a. Who does what in the house? Is this mutually satisfactory?
    b. Who makes decisions? How are they made? Is there mutual discussion?
    c. What are the changes that members would like?

    d. How do the parents see their roles being changed with a new infant?

2. How do members usually define situations that happen?
    a. Does the family generally consolidate in times of trouble?
    b. Do they tend to be optimistic, pessimistic, or do attitudes vary with situations?
    c. What are the communication patterns? Who talks to whom? Do problems usually get solved with discussion?

3. What are the family's material and emotional resources?
    a. Is the environment safe and healthful?
    Is housing safe and adequate? Is there appropriate room for the expected infant? If not, what plans are being made to remedy the situation? Is the housing environment structured to prevent accidents? If not, what remedy is planned?
    b. Is the family healthful?
    What is the general health status of the family? Have there been or are there now illnesses? If so, has appropriate medical (or dental) care been sought? Is there a regular source of medical and dental care for the family? Does the woman use maternity services appropriately? If not, why not? How does the family usually pay for health services? Is health insurance or a health maintenance organization (HMO) service available? What are the family's usual health habits (exercise, rest, nutrition, smoking, substance abuse)?
    c. Are finances adequate? Who contributes? Will the pregnancy make a difference?
    d. Who turns to whom for emotional support? Who is the woman's main support at this time? Who is the man's main support at this time?

4. Are there interpersonal or intrapersonal difficulties?
    a. Are there long-term problems? What are the attempts to resolve them?
    b. Are there problems specific to this pregnancy?
    c. What alternatives for solution for the existing problems do the parents see?

5. What are the specific plans for the baby and for themselves during pregnancy?
    a. What are their plans for themselves as parents?
    b. What are their plans for the infant?
    c. Are siblings anticipated (if this is the first child)?
    d. What are the plans for siblings?

NURSING CARE PLAN

EARLY UNCOMPLICATED PREGNANCY

Goals (expected outcomes)	Intervention	Rationale	Evaluation
ANXIETY—RELATED TO ADAPTATIONS TO PREGNANCY			
Client or couple will demonstrate behaviors that are indicative of acceptance of the pregnancy and of planning for the pregnancy.	Establish rapport by providing caring, unhurried environment in which couple experiences openness to express their feelings and concerns. Provide opportunity for client or couple to ask questions of concern when they arrive for visit. Answer questions client or couple may have as health history and cultural and family assessment data are obtained.	Helps decrease stress by promoting opportunity to explore feelings and to have questions answered.	Client or couple verbalizes understanding of facts related to diagnosis of pregnancy. Client or couple expresses knowledge of appropriate methods of adaptation to current concerns.

FAMILY COPING: POTENTIAL FOR GROWTH—RELATED TO PLANNING AND PREPARATION FOR INFANT

Client or couple will explore role changes associated with pregnancy.	Provide opportunity to explore methods of resolving extrafamilial stressors.	Reduces stressors so client or couple can concentrate on role adaptations related to pregnancy.	Client or couple demonstrates progress in resolving stressors.
Client or couple will demonstrate behaviors that are indicative of a smooth transition as a growing family.	Provide information about community support services if assistance is needed in resolving intrafamilial stressors.		Client or couple becomes involved in activities (uses resources) that promote role adaptation.
	Provide information about community resources that help promote positive adaptation to pregnancy and positive outcomes of pregnancy (e.g., pregnangyms, childbirth education classes, sibling preparation classes, baby care classes).	Helps to prepare for childbirth experience. Promotes sense of wellbeing. Encourages active involvement of self and family members. Promotes sense of selfworth.	Client or couple verbalizes recognition of pregnancy as real.
	Provide literature for the expectant couple.		

Continued

NURSING CARE PLAN

EARLY UNCOMPLICATED PREGNANCY—continued

Goals (expected outcomes)	Intervention	Rationale	Evaluation
FAMILY COPING: POTENTIAL FOR GROWTH—RELATED TO PLANNING AND PREPARATION FOR INFANT—cont'd			
	Provide information from examination findings that suggest confirmation of pregnancy.	Promotes initial bonding as moves through stages of accepting tentative pregnancy as actual pregnancy.	
KNOWLEDGE DEFICIT—REGARDING SELF-CARE DURING PREGNANCY			
Client or couple will demonstrate new knowledge by using health practices that will promote a healthy mother and infant.	Answer questions and clarify misunderstandings and misinformation.	Practices arising from incorrect knowledge may be harmful to woman and developing fetus. Correct information promotes safe practices and a sense of positiveness about self-care.	Client or couple uses self-care practices that promote positive physiologic responses to pregnancy. Client or couple blends cultural beliefs with behaviors that promote a healthy pregnancy and neonate.

Continued

Explain schedule for return visits and assessments and explain care that will be provided during visit.	Promotes confidence in caregivers. Reinforces interest of caregivers in client or couple. Reinforces importance of continuous care throughout pregnancy.
Provide anticipatory guidance by giving information that promotes positive adaptations and self-care practices (e.g., exercise, employment, hygienic measures, sexual practices, medication).	Understanding of self-care activities promotes a sense of individual responsibility and interest in achieving expectations.
Provide information about teratogens (e.g., environmental substances, licit and illicit drugs, certain infections.)	The first trimester of fetal development is essential to positive neonatal outcomes. Couple's awareness of effect of teratogens may promote positive health practices.

Nursing Care Plan

Early Uncomplicated Pregnancy—continued

Goals (expected outcomes)	Intervention	Rationale	Evaluation
KNOWLEDGE DEFICIT—REGARDING SELF-CARE DURING PREGNANCY—cont'd			
	Encourage client or couple to write down questions that arise between visits so that they can be addressed at next visit.	Demonstrates interests in client or couple and promotes client's active participation in own care.	
ALTERED NUTRITION: LESS THAN BODY REQUIREMENTS—RELATED TO NAUSEA AND VOMITING ASSOCIATED WITH EARLY PREGNANCY			
Client reports reduction in nausea and vomiting and evidences a weight gain of 3 pounds by the end of the first trimester.	Teach to eat foods high in carbohydrates (soda crackers, dry toast) before arising. Teach to eat six small meals per day. Provide information about nutritional needs of mother and fetus.	Decreases gastric acidity, thus reducing nausea and vomiting. Prevents malnutrition and dehydration, which compromise fetal development and physiologic adaptation essential to a healthy pregnancy.	Client is able to retain dry carbohydrate on arising. Client adjusts dietary intake to promote retention of food.

Chapter 2

NUTRITION IN PREGNANCY

Nutrition plays a key role in the outcome of pregnancy. A woman's nutritional status during the pregnancy helps to determine her health and well-being and that of her child. The following tools will assist you in helping the pregnant woman understand why nutrition is so important.

NUTRITIONAL AND DIETARY GUIDELINES

1. Include client's family, when appropriate, in nutritional planning.
2. Incorporate client's food choices and preferences in the nutritional plan.
3. Assist client to increase her knowledge of needed nutrients.
4. Encourage and reinforce correct choices and willingness to make adaptations.
5. Provide firm guidance when indicated.
6. Document dietary counseling sessions, including printed materials and client's understanding of information.

COMPONENTS OF WEIGHT GAIN DURING PREGNANCY

	lb
Fetal components	
Fetus	7½
Placenta	1½
Amniotic fluid	2¼
Maternal components	
Uterus and breasts	3½
Blood	4½
Extracellular fluid	3½
Other tissue (fat)	1¾

RECOMMENDED DIETARY ALLOWANCES FOR ADULT WOMEN (AGES 25 TO 50 YEARS)

	Nonpregnant	Pregnant
Energy (kcal)	2200	+300
Protein (gm)	50	60
Vitamin A (RE)	800	800
Vitamin D (μg)	5	10
Vitamin E (mg)	8	10
Vitamin C (ascorbic acid) (mg)	60	70
Folic acid (μg)	180	+400
Niacin (mg)	15	17
Riboflavin (mg)	1.3	1.6
Thiamin (mg)	1.1	1.5
Vitamin B_6 (mg)	1.6	2.2
Vitamin B_{12} (μg)	2.0	2.2
Calcium (mg)	800	1200
Phosphorus (mg)	800	1200
Iodine (μg)	150	175
Iron (mg)	15	*30
Magnesium (mg)	280	320
Zinc (mg)	12	15

From Food and Nutrition Board, Subcommittee on the Tenth Edition of the Recommended Dietary Allowances, 10 ed. Washington, DC, National Academy Press, 1989.
* 30-60 mg of supplemental iron per day is recommended.

RECOMMENDED CALORIE INTAKE

	Age (years) or condition	Calories per day
Females	11-14	2200
	15-18	2200
	19-24	2200
	25-50	2200
	51 +	1900
Pregnant	1st trimester	+0
	2nd trimester	+300
	3rd trimester	+300
Lactating	1st 6 months	+500
	2nd 6 months	+500

RECOMMENDED PROTEIN INTAKE

Nutrient	Amount (set by National Research Council)		Reasons for increased nutrient need in pregnancy	Food sources
	Nonpregnant adult need (age 19 to 24)	Pregnancy need		
Protein	46 g	76 to 160 g	Rapid fetal tissue growth	Milk
			Amniotic fluid	Cheese
			Placenta growth and development	Eggs
				Meats
			Maternal tissue growth: uterus, breasts	Grains
				Legumes
			Increased maternal circulating blood volume, hemoglobin increase, plasma protein increase	Nuts
			Maternal storage reserves for labor, delivery, and lactation	

From Bininger C et al: American Nursing Review for NCLEX-RN. Springhouse, Pa, Springhouse, 1989.

NUTRITIONAL RISK FACTORS

Category	Factor	Significance
Age	Adolescence	Increased nutritional needs; possible poor food habits; noncompliance
	Older gravidas	Possible increased incidence of other risk factors
Obstetric history	High parity or frequent conceptions	Depletion of maternal nutrient stores
	Previous obstetric complications	Possible nutritional relationship may recur
Medical history	Preexisting medical problems	May affect ingestion, utilization, or absorption of nutrients
Complications of current pregnancy	Development of complications such as, anemia, preeclampsia, or gestational diabetes	Development of nutritional deficiencies due to increased nutritional needs
Maternal weight	Low prepregnancy weight	Increased incidence of pregnancy and neonatal complications
	Insufficient weight gain	Indication of poor maternal and fetal nutrition; increased number of low-birth-weight infants
	Obesity	Possible poor nutritional habits; increased incidence of pregnancy complications
	Excessive weight gain	If sudden, may indicate preeclampsia; lack of agreement on other possible risks

Dysfunctional dietary patterns	Dietary faddism	Diets often inadequate to meet fetal or maternal nutritional needs
	Pica	Displacement of nutritious foods, often related to iron deficiency anemia
	Excessive use of alcohol, drugs, or tobacco	Interference with appetite and with utilization of some nutrients
Socioeconomic status	Low income	Limited ability to buy sufficient food; possible chronic malnutrition
Cultural or ethnic group	Ethnic or language differences	Interference with ability to find usual foods; misinterpretation of dietary instructions
	Herbal remedies	Allergies, abortifacient effect
Psychologic conditions	Depression, anorexia nervosa	Possible reduced caloric and nutrient intake

POSSIBLE ADVERSE EFFECTS OF POOR NUTRITION DURING THE REPRODUCTIVE CYCLE*

Reproductive problems
  Infertility
  Abortion
  Stillbirth
  Neonatal death

Pregnancy problems
  Maternal anemias
  Vitamin deficiencies
  Preeclampsia and eclampsia
  Placental abnormalities
  Gestational diabetes
  Vitamin deficiencies
  Pica-related complications
  Dystocia
  Lactation difficulties
  Slow postpartum maternal recovery

Neonatal problems
  Low-birth-weight infants
  Delayed mental and physical
    development of infant
  Congenital malformations
  Fetal alcohol syndrome
  Neonatal anemias
  Vitamin deficiencies

---

*Obviously many other factors influence the occurrence of these problems, but prepregnant status and nutritional status and nutrient intake during pregnancy play a significant role.

GUIDE TO HEMATOLOGIC LABORATORY TESTS

Test	Nonpregnant normal values	Deficiency
Ferritin (μg/l)	40-160	≤ 12
Serum Iron (μg/dl)	65-165	<42
Transferrin (TIBC) (μg/dl)	300-360	>400
% Saturation	25-40	<15-20
Mean corpuscular volume (MCV) (fl)	82-92	<80 (iron) >96 (folate)
Mean corpuscular hemoglobin concentration (MCHC) (%)	32-36	<32
Mean corpuscular hemoglobin (MCH) (pg)	27-31	<27
Protoporphyrin (μg/dl RBC)	30	>100

From Dimperio D: Florida's Guide to Maternal Nutrition. Tallahassee, State of Florida, Department of Health and Rehabilitation Services, 1986.

EVALUATION OF LABORATORY TESTS

Laboratory tests are used to determine the presence and level of various nutrients. These tests can identify or confirm specific nutrient-related problems. Special attention is given to hemoglobin and hematocrit results as these two measurements reflect nutritional status. Hematologic laboratory tests also are important diagnostic tools for identifying iron and folate deficiences.

SAMPLE NARRATIVE CHARTING

16 wks' gestation. Wt: 105. Gained 1 lb past 4 wks (see weight gain grid); Hgb: 10; Hct: 32. Easily fatigued; no energy; looks tired, pale. Discussed 24-hr diet record, chronic fatigue, food budget and transportation problems, noncompliance with pamphlet "Food for You." Stressed need for additional calories, iron, increased protein for her and fetus. 3200 calorie diet, sample meal given and discussed; Rx for Natafort Filmseal with instructions; verbalized understanding of dosage, side effects, nursing considerations. Verbalized understanding of diet and vitamins but needs assistance for buying both. Referred to nutritionist to plan meals, WIC for eligibility (pamphlet given). Instructed to make appt. this week; verbalized compliance. To submit 3-day diet diary for review; recheck wt., counseling in follow-up visit × 2 wks. Requested report from nutritionist prior to next visit. Repeat Hgb, Hct × 4 weeks. Will refer to Dr. Jones for work-up pending results.

NURSING CARE PLAN

INSUFFICIENT WEIGHT GAIN

Goals (expected outcomes)	Interventions	Rationale	Evaluation
ALTERED NUTRITION: LESS THAN BODY REQUIREMENTS—RELATED TO INADEQUATE DIETARY INTAKE			
Client will maintain adequate prenatal nutritional status and meet energy demands of pregnancy effectively.	Explain physiologic demands of pregnancy and need for increased caloric intake.	Increased maternal metabolic rate and fetal growth require large amounts of energy. Calories provide energy for maternal body processes, thermal balance, physical activity, and for building and maintaining maternal and fetal/placental tissue. Nutrients are vital to growth and maintenance of healthy tissue and for effective function of body processes.	Client exhibits expected pattern of weight gain throughout the pregnancy: First trimester: 1 to 4 pounds Second trimester: 10 to 12 pounds. Third trimester: 10 to 12 pounds. No complaints of fatigue or lack of energy to perform normal activities.

KNOWLEDGE DEFICIT—REGARDING NUTRITIONAL NEEDS IN PREGNANCY

Client will explain benefits of high caloric and nutrient intake during pregnancy. Identify foods high in protein, vitamins, and iron and list foods high in "empty" calories.

Discuss dietary requirements during pregnancy. Emphasize relationship to maternal and fetal health.

Poor maternal nutrition is associated with a higher incidence of: complicated pregnancy (e.g., spontaneous abortion, intrauterine fetal growth retardation, stillbirth), reduced fetal brain cell development, and developmental lags in infancy.

Increases client's understanding of the importance of eating a well-balanced, high protein, high caloric diet during pregnancy. Facilitates compliance with dietary management.

Client requests pamphlets to take home and denies cultural taboos or influence on food choices or eating habits.

Refer to nutritionist for meal planning, menus; WIC for eligibility for food buying assistance.

Increases potential for compliance with dietary management.

Client reports appointments with WIC; using food checks to purchase food and vitamins.

Continued

NURSING CARE PLAN

INSUFFICIENT WEIGHT GAIN—continued

Goals (expected outcomes)	Interventions	Rationale	Evaluation
KNOWLEDGE DEFICIT—REGARDING NUTRITIONAL NEEDS IN PREGNANCY—cont'd			
	Distribute and discuss "Food for You," and "What is WIC" pamphlets. Assist in identifying acceptable substitutes for foods disliked or not tolerated well, e.g., milk and milk products.		Client presents own menus developed with assistance of nutritionist. Daily dietary record verifies compliance with recommendations; reveals 3200 calories, 16% protein (76 g). Client reports taking prenatal supplements (vitamins, iron, folic acid) as directed for individual management and denies pica. Hemoglobin and hematocrit remain within acceptable limits. Hemoglobin: 10 g or more Hematocrit: >35%

Chapter 3

Prenatal Education

Prenatal education is an essential component of family-centered maternity care. It prepares the pregnant woman and her support person for the physical and emotional experiences of childbearing. This chapter presents information essential to the assessment, goals, and interventions needed to ensure the expectant couple's willingness to learn and understand the birthing process.

RELAXATION

SUGGESTIONS FOR PROMOTING RELAXATION

Before beginning a relaxation exercise:
1. Provide a calm, relaxed environment with quiet music.
2. Make sure you will not be interrupted during the exercise.
3. Empty your bladder.
4. Assume a comfortable position with all limbs supported with pillows.

CLIENT SELF-CARE EDUCATION

THE ROLE OF THE COACH IN RELAXATION

Action

1. Make a visual check of your partner's position.

2. During the exercises check your partner periodically for relaxation by picking up her arm.

3. If you note any tension, relax it away by using a light massage on the tense part and verbally reminding her to relax.

Rationale

1. Signs of tension include frowning, rigid neck and shoulders, and clenched fists.

2. If she has achieved a state of relaxation, the upper arm, lower arm, and wrist should move separately and feel heavy in your hands. She should not move or lift her arm for you.

3. Verbal communication reminds the mother that she is tense. The touch communication identifies area of tension.

CLIENT SELF-CARE EDUCATION

EVENTS TAKING PLACE DURING LABOR AND DELIVERY PROCESS

Typical changes in mother	Helpful comfort measures	Typical care provider activities
FIRST-STAGE LABOR: ONSET—2 CM DILATATION		
Physical		
Contractions mild, 5-30 minutes apart, 30-40 seconds long; may be felt in front or as backache	Continue some normal activities, but include rest or naps.	Health care provider contacted; plans discussed
Pinkish vaginal discharge; bag of waters may break; diarrhea common	If hungry, eat light, easily digested foods.	
Psychologic		
Combination of anxiety and excitement	Practice mind and muscle relaxation with contractions.	
Social		
Wants to make contact with those who are to be with her at birth	Calmly finish packing and making last-minute arrangements.	

FIRST-STAGE LABOR: 2-4 CM DILATION

Physical

Contractions range from 3 to 30 minutes apart, 25-45 seconds long Typically mild, somewhat irregular, but progressively stronger and closer	Make her comfortable; encourage walking and sitting. Check into planned birth site after discussion with birth attendant. When appropriate, provide diversion, such as music, card games.	Checks contractions for frequency, duration, and strength Checks blood pressure, temperature, fetal heart rate, urine protein, blood type
May be experienced as ache or pressure in low back, menstrual cramps, pressure or tightening in pubic area		Provides information on progress to mother, family, and other caregivers
Mother stops walking or talking through contractions at approximately 4 cm dilation		Completes admission procedures such as history; performs enema and/or shave when indicated

Psychologic

Typically comfortable, smiling, excited, ready for labor experience	Observe response to contractions; check relaxation and breathing.	Becomes acquainted with mother and family and tells them what to expect
May show anxiety through tears or talkativeness; may gasp for breath, make fists and rocking motion	Encourage mother not to start breathing techniques too soon; emphasize relaxation. Listen closely; praise efforts.	Encourages mother's participation in decisions about her care

Adapted from Humenick S: Your labor guide. Lamaze Parents Magazine, 1989, pp 72-77.

Continued

EVENTS TAKING PLACE DURING LABOR AND DELIVERY PROCESS—continued

Typical changes in mother	Helpful comfort measures	Typical care provider activities
FIRST-STAGE LABOR: 2-4 CM DILATATION—cont'd		
Social		
Typically sociable, interested in what is going on, asking questions, reporting symptoms, enjoying diversion	Accept behavior.	Observes support of family/friends and encourages them to provide help and company
	Provide privacy if desired by mother for vaginal examinations or other procedures.	
May or may not want family member present during admission procedures	Provide entertainment and company as desired by mother.	
FIRST-STAGE LABOR: 5-7 CM DILATATION		
Physical		
Contractions range from 2-5 minutes apart, 40-60 seconds duration; stronger intensity, longer peaks, and becoming more uncomfortable and annoying	Support mother's desires through assistance with relaxation and breathing patterns; remind her of focal point; add effleurage (finger-tip massage).	Continues assessment of infant heart rate, blood pressure, dilation, and contractions
		Straightens sheets and changes pads to increase comfort

May experience dry mouth, nausea or vomiting, diaphoresis (perspiration), diarrhea	Anticipate physical needs; encourage hourly urination; offer lip balm, ice chips, position changes, cool damp cloth to forehead as desired, or hot towels to areas of discomfort.
May appear flushed or pale; if unprepared, may breathe deeply, rapidly, or unevenly and may hyperventilate (experienced as dizziness or tingling of lips or fingers)	Rub back or apply counterpressure to lower back as desired by mother. Try pelvic rocking; encourage position changes.	Provides medication requested as an adjunct to support, rather than a substitute for it; considers mother-baby safety as well as mother's desires

Psychologic

If she tires, may become more restless, less relaxed, and uncertain of her ability to cope	Keep mother informed between contractions; use simple, short phrases.	Encourages family support; teaches and supplements labor support as appropriate
May moan or cry		

Social

Typically more serious; less talkative, attentive, and able to understand	Someone should stay with mother. Family members should eat and take rests to prepare themselves for the birth; ask for nurse or other family member to substitute during breaks.	Assists family members in meeting their own needs for breaks, foods, comfort
Desires companionship		
Easily upset by restriction, assessment procedures, or even attempts to support her		

Continued

EVENTS TAKING PLACE DURING LABOR AND DELIVERY PROCESS—continued

Typical changes in mother	Helpful comfort measures	Typical care provider activities
FIRST-STAGE LABOR: 8-10 CM DILATATION		
Physical		
Contractions range from 1-3 minutes apart, 50-90 seconds long, peaking almost immediately, frequently with double peaks and urge to push	Provide cool sponging of face or warm blankets as needed. Provide firm low back pressure or back rub as desired.	Continues assessment of infant heart rate, blood pressure, dilatation, station, position Avoids new medications since the worst is nearly over for the mother and it is not desirable to give medications close to infant's birth; strong coaching should get mother through this difficult but brief part
Typically perspires; increased vaginal discharge	Instruct to pace breathing if nauseated, possibly breathing into a paper sack.	
May have severe low backache, hiccoughing, belching, nausea or vomiting, shaking of upper thighs, pulling sensation in pelvis, cramps in legs, buttocks	Encourage appropriate breathing to prevent pushing if the urge to push occurs too early.	
Bag of waters may break		
Drowsy between contractions		
Psychologic		
Typically less responsive; indecisive, restless, and irritable; loses perspective	Work with her in a calm, organized manner. Stay with her. Provide strong coaching with establishment of eye-to-eye contact when instructing.	
If awakened during a contraction, she may be unable to cope effectively with that contraction		

Often feels unable to go on
Natural amnesia; may not remember much of this part

Social
Totally focused on self
Desires constant companionship

Anticipate contraction with palpation or clock and wake mother, helping her begin breathing and other coping strategies. Let her sleep between contractions if she can arouse before contractions.

Provide perspective, encouragement. This is the most difficult part, but often lasts only 12-20 contractions.

SECOND-STAGE LABOR: BIRTH

Physical
Contractions less frequent, every 2-5 minutes, 45-90 seconds long
Rectal bulging, flattening of perineum, bloody show
Becomes awake, alert, gets "second wind," usually has strong urge to push with contraction unless regional block such as epidural given

Assist in pushing with contractions by getting her into an advantageous position such as an upright position where gravity can help.
Help her avoid excessive breath holding during pushing by having her let a small amount of air escape from her mouth while pushing with abdominal muscles and relaxing pelvic muscles.

Encourages coaching from family, instructs them, helps them accept her behavior; gives her support and provides companionship
Allows mother to try pushing a few times before urging a decision on anesthesia
Especially if second stage progress is slow, encourages mother to experiment with positions such as squatting if appropriate

Continued

EVENTS TAKING PLACE DURING LABOR AND DELIVERY PROCESS—continued

Typical changes in mother	Helpful comfort measures	Typical care provider activities
SECOND-STAGE LABOR: BIRTH—cont'd		
Pushing with contractions felt as a great relief; also accompanied by sensations of stretching, burning, and "splitting" until baby moves down and creates a natural anesthesia	Encourage her to take a new breath every 5 to 6 seconds while maintaining abdominal pressure. This avoids drops in infant heartbeat, which can occur with prolonged breath holding.	Continues to check infant heart rate and blood pressure, especially if mother has had an epidural or saddle
Could find pushing painful if mother fails to relax pelvic floor or if infant's head is still rotating		
Psychologic		
May panic, especially if unprepared; first attempts at pushing often uncoordinated	Keep someone at mother's head during birth to avoid all eyes on her bottom.	Explains birth procedures as they occur
		Provides mirror for birth if desired

Social
Likely to be totally involved during contractions but eager for interaction between contractions; desirous of family presence especially if there are complications

| | Encourage, stay with mother. | Avoids situations where mother is asked to blow instead of push because she must wait for staff |

THIRD STAGE AND RECOVERY

Physical

Contractions temporarily cease with infant birth, then resume	If infant will breast-feed, mother should offer breast during first hours. Healthy infants are typically awake and alert.	For infant, provides care, observes, footprints
Detachment of placenta accompanied by upward rise of uterus in abdomen		For mother, continues to monitor her blood pressure and bleeding; assists in urinating; covers with warm blankets; teaches to massage own uterus; evaluates need for medication
Recovery period accompanied by vaginal bleeding, shaking, chills, bladder filling; uterus should stay firm but may relax, increasing bleeding		

Continued

EVENTS TAKING PLACE DURING LABOR AND DELIVERY PROCESS—continued

Typical changes in mother	Helpful comfort measures	Typical care provider activities
THIRD STAGE AND RECOVERY—cont'd		
Psychologic		
Asks questions about labor and delivery events, recalls events vividly, may feel apologetic for labor behavior	Reassure regarding acceptance of labor behavior with no apology needed.	Explains details of birth experience as desired
Seeks reassurance that infant is normal	Praise regarding labor accomplishment.	Explains recovery routines
May be very alert or may want to sleep		Plans to visit the next day to allow mother to review labor and birth events
Social		
Typically alert, happy, tired, expressing feelings through talking, laughing, and/or crying	Share experiences and feelings. Spend time with infant; begin process of becoming a family.	Delays administration of medication to infant's eyes until after family has been together
Seeks contact with infant		Encourages mother-father-infant interaction through touching, cuddling, breast-feeding
Expresses feelings with family		

RELAXATION TECHNIQUES

Name and type	Description	Feedback
Progressive relaxation (modifies muscular responses)	Consists of systematically tensing and releasing muscles; developed by Edmond Jacobson, modified by J. Wolpe into a 6-week approach with home practice.	Primary feedback initially described as the awareness of participant who focuses on the sensation of tensing and relaxing each muscle. Either a coach or electromyograph can provide feedback.
Neuromuscular dissociation (modifies muscular responses)	Follows progressive relaxation by asking the participant to tense some muscles and relax others simultaneously; introduced in this country by Elisabeth Bing.	Feedback by having the coach check relaxation and tension was introduced by Karmel and Bing—not mentioned in books by either Fernand Lamaze or Irwin Chabon.
Autogenic training (mental control modifying muscular and autonomic systems responses)	Training through suggestions including "my right arm is heavy" or "my left arm is warm"; includes slowing the heart and respiration and cooling the forehead; developed by J. Schultz and W. Luther.	Feedback initially described as the awareness of the participant with no outside feedback; has been used with biofeedback equipment, thermometers.

Continued

From Humenick S: Teaching relaxation. Childbirth Educator, Summer 1984.

RELAXATION TECHNIQUES—continued

Name and type	Description	Feedback
Meditation (modifies vascular and neurotransmitter responses)	Defined by Herbert Benson as dwelling on an object (repeating a sound or gazing at an object) while emptying all thoughts and distractions in a quiet atmosphere in a comfortable position; used in transcendental meditation and yoga.	Concentration on a focal point and on breathing patterns would be forms of meditation by Benson's definition. Participant can monitor self but also receives coach's feedback on both activities.
Visual imagery	Includes techniques such as visualizing oneself on a warm beach or as a bag of cement or going down a staircase; often precedes introduction of other kinds of relaxation; may also be used to visualize and potentially affect specific body parts as in cancer therapy; may be used in desensitization in which one relaxes while visualizing a potentially threatening situation; used in labor rehearsals.	

Touching/massaging	Touch has always been a way for one person to calm another. There is evidence of actual transfer of energy taking place in some forms of touching. In childbirth preparation touching is associated with muscular relaxation (Sheila Kissinger).	Feedback from coach includes informing when muscle tension is felt, necessitating advanced coaching. Coaches may need first to discern relaxation by moving a limb.
Biofeedback	Electromyograph measures neuromuscular tension. Thermometer measures skin temperature at extremities. Galvanic skin reflex records conductivity changes because of the action of sweat glands at the surface of the skin. Electroencephalograph distinguishes alpha, beta, and theta waves in the brain.	Feedback from all of these machines is in one or more of these forms: visualization of a meter, listening to a sound, or watching a set of flashing lights.

BREATHING TECHNIQUES

1. Slow paced breathing
   This is relaxed breathing at a slower rate than usual. You may use your nose or mouth to inhale or exhale, whichever is more comfortable. Slow paced breathing provides good oxygenation and is conducive to relaxation.
   Practice guide
   Always begin and end your practice contractions with a cleansing breath. As you practice slow paced breathing, find a focal point; as you breathe, count "in 2, 3, 4—out 2, 3, 4," to keep your pace slow.
   Practice "having" contractions of varying lengths, beginning with a simulated 30- or 45-second contraction and increasing the length as you progress to the other breathing techniques.
   After you have mastered slow paced breathing, you may move on to modified paced breathing.

2. Modified paced breathing
   This is breathing at a slightly faster rate than usual. The breaths are shallow, and hyperventilation is possible if you breathe too rapidly. Begin slowly with the contraction and increase the pace with the intensity of the contraction.
   Practice guide
   a. Breathe in a manner that is most comfortable for you so you can concentrate on the diversional activity of the breathing rather than on feeling as though it is an effort to breathe.
   Breathe at a pace no faster than two times your normal respiratory rate taking shallow breaths. Be aware of signs of hyperventilation (dizziness, light-headedness, and tingling around the mouth and in the hands) and the corrective measures (cupping hands over nose and mouth and rebreathing the exhaled air, or breathing into a paper bag).
   During the practice session your coach should be observing you for signs of tension (frowning, rigid neck and shoulders, clenched fists). He or she should make sure you are aware of tension and help you relax.

3. Pattern paced breathing
   a. This is performed at the same rate as modified paced breathing, but a soft blow is added at regular intervals to create a rhythmic pattern. This technique requires much concentration and is valuable in the more active stages of labor.

Practice guide

The coach gives verbal cues that create the breathing pattern. For example, he or she selects a number between one and four, which is the number of breaths the woman will take, followed by a short blow. The coach then selects another number.

The numbers, or pattern, should be varied so the mother's concentration focuses on the breathing rather than on the contraction.

b. This alternate pattern, using one breath and one blow, can counteract the desire to push.

Practice guide

To practice for a premature urge to push, the coach gives a cue that the urge to push is felt. The woman then uses a panting type breathing to control the urge.

4. Pushing

This technique assists in delivering the baby.

Practice guide

Begin the contraction with two cleansing breaths. Take a third breath and hold it for a count of six while exerting downward force with your abdominal muscles. When you need more air, take a quick breath and repeat the process until the contraction is over. End the contraction with a cleansing breath. Be sure the muscles used in Kegel exercises are relaxed as you are pushing.

SUGGESTIONS FOR PRACTICING BREATHING TECHNIQUES

When practicing the breathing techniques, always remember the following:

1. The breathing techniques do not work alone; relaxation is the key component to success.
2. Always begin with slow paced breathing because it provides a physiologic calming effect and decreases the impact of stressors. After that the breathing techniques do not have to be used in any prescribed order. Use the breathing techniques that best promote control during labor.
3. Coaches also need to practice all the breathing techniques with their partner to assist the mother with getting the pattern. Time should be set aside for the coach and mother to practice together.

4. Breathing should be practiced in a calm, relaxing environment with quiet music. Use music that you enjoy. You will develop an awareness of the music and an association with relaxation that can be beneficial in labor.
5. Develop an awareness of breathing.
   a. When practicing the relaxation exercises, pay attention to your rate and depth of breathing.
   b. Use a cleansing breath by breathing in slowly and deeply through the nose and out slowly through the mouth to promote relaxation.
   c. Notice how different positions affect your breathing and use this information during labor.

ASSESSMENT

FOCUS ASSESSMENT

Identify readiness to learn.
    Identify couple's expectations of the training program.
    Determine couple's current knowledge regarding self-care techniques for stress management.
Explore their usual methods of coping with stressful situations.
Observe the couple's patterns of interaction and decision making, i.e., interactions with each other, nurse-instructor, and other couples. Note evidence of dominance or mutual support.
Identify areas where individualized teaching and support is needed.
    Note type of questions asked, response to teaching methods, and participation in learning activities.

NURSING CARE PLAN

COUPLES PARTICIPATING IN TRAINING FOR RELAXATION FOR PREGNANCY/LABOR AND BIRTH/LIFE STRESS

Goals (expected outcomes)	Interventions	Rationale	Evaluation
KNOWLEDGE DEFICIT—REGARDING RELAXATION SKILLS			
Client will demonstrate relaxation techniques and state their benefits in everyday life and for reducing labor pain.	After determining what woman and partner know, explain other benefits of relaxation. Include benefits for right now, labor and birth, and later life. Give other examples in everyday life that may be familiar, e.g., "tension headache" (tension causes increased pain).	Client can easily relate relaxation techniques to everyday occurrences.	Client verbalizes understanding. May contribute some benefits. No further questions.
NONCOMPLIANCE—RELATED TO PARTNER'S LACK OF KNOWLEDGE ABOUT IMPORTANCE OF RELAXATION SKILLS			
The partner will be able to participate in and understand the need for relaxation exercises.	Include partner in teaching when possible. Discuss health benefit for partner also. Have partner participate by doing relaxation with woman as you teach.	Partner, as part of the team, is instrumental in having the client achieve a state of relaxation.	Partner assists with woman's learning, practice, and evaluation; gives appropriate feedback during practice.

Continued

NURSING CARE PLAN

COUPLES PARTICIPATING IN TRAINING FOR RELAXATION FOR PREGNANCY/LABOR AND BIRTH/LIFE STRESS—continued

Goals (expected outcomes)	Interventions	Rationale	Evaluation
NONCOMPLIANCE—RELATED TO PARTNER'S LACK OF KNOWLEDGE ABOUT IMPORTANCE OF RELAXATION SKILLS—cont'd			
	Teach partner how to assess woman's level of relaxation and how to give positive nonjudgmental feedback to her.		Couple practices, evidenced by verbal reports and by woman's increasing ability to relax as observed by nurse during practice sessions:
	Explain it will take time and daily practice (15-20 min) to be effective in labor/stress.	Partner may mutually benefit from relaxation techniques.	Relaxed jaw Slow, regular breathing Smoothed facial muscles Legs rolled out and feet at 45 degree angle to each other
	Motivate by making sure couple understands benefits and physiologic consequences resulting from unnecessary tension. Help couple plan specific home practice schedule with self-reward system to help motivate.		Couple acts as team during observed practice session.

MATERNAL NURSING CARE

Chapter 4

OBSTETRIC ANALGESIA AND ANESTHESIA

Pain is whatever the experiencing person says it is. The quality of labor discomfort (pain) is difficult to describe. Any painful sensation can have various qualities, including burning, prickling, aching, sharpness or "shooting". Pain can be deep or superficial. Words commonly used by women in labor to describe their pain are sharp, cramping, aching, throbbing, stabbing, hot, shooting, heavy, exhausting, intense, and tight.

Clients describe the pain during delivery as pressure, stretching, splitting, or burning of the vaginal and perineal areas.

This chapter presents information on nonpharmacologic methods of analgesia and the various anesthetics used for labor pain relief.

NURSING GUIDELINES FOR PAIN RELIEF MEASURES

Use a variety of pain relief measures.

Use pain relief measures *before* pain becomes severe. (It is easier to prevent severe pain and panic than to alleviate them once they occur.)

Include those pain relief measures that the client believes will be effective.

Take into account the client's ability to be active or passive in the application of the pain relief measure.

Regarding the potency of the pain relief measure needed, rely on the client's experience of the severity of pain rather than the known physical stimuli.

If a pain relief measure is ineffective the first time it is used during a contraction, encourage the client to try it at least one or two more times before abandoning it.

DISTRACTION TECHNIQUES

Concentrating on a focal point (staring at an object during a contraction)

Tapping out the rhythm of a song

Performing rhythmic head movements

Using a rhythmic breathing pattern while concentrating on relaxation

Concentrating on imagery (thinking the infant down and out)

Changing positions and massaging the abdomen (effleurage)

Using breathing techniques

LEGAL AND ETHICAL CONSIDERATIONS

One of the most important responsibilities of the nurse in Labor and Delivery is the careful monitoring of maternal and fetal status as indicated by the criteria below.

Liability for negligence in the labor and delivery period generally centers around the failure to attend to the client or to monitor the progress of the fetus during labor. The American College of Obstetricians/Gynecologists (ACOG) recommends that auscultation of the fetal heart be done at 15 to 30 minute intervals during the active phase of first stage of labor and at 5 to 15 minute intervals during second stage of labor for high-risk and low-risk clients respectively. Evaluation of the FHR information when continuous electronic monitoring is done may take place at the intervals suggested for auscultation or more frequently depending on the individual client-care situation. Written documentation is also in accordance with institutional policy and procedure. The length, duration, and intensity of uterine contractions should be palpated or monitored. These periodic monitorings must be recorded. The court views an item that was not documented as one that was not done.[*]

---

[*]The information given in this paragraph was adapted from Northrup C, Kelly M: Legal Issues in Nursing. St. Louis, CV Mosby, 1987 and from The Organization of Obstetric, Gynecologic and Neonatal Nurses: Nursing Responsibilities in Implementing Intrapartum Fetal Heart Rate Monitoring. NAACOG, 1988.

COMMON MEDICATIONS USED FOR ANALGESIA DURING LABOR

Drug	Category	Dosage and route	Actions	Comments
Meperidine hydrochloride (Demerol)	Narcotic: a nonopiate, addicting analgesic	IM: 50-100 mg, repeated 3-4 hr prn IV: 25 mg, repeated 1-2 hr prn	Peaks IM: Onset 10 min Peaks 60 min Duration 2-3 hr IV: Onset 5 min Duration 1-2 hr	Maternal effects: analgesia, sedation, nausea, vomiting Fetal effects: loss of variability of fetal heart tone; can cause respiratory depression at birth; can cause decreased muscle tone at birth
Butorphanol tartrate (Stadol)	Nonnarcotic analgesic	IM: 2 mg repeated 3-4 hr prn IV: 1 mg repeated 3-4 hr prn	Peaks IM: Onset 10 min Peaks 30-60 min Duration 1-4 hr IV: More rapid onset and peak	Maternal effects: sedation, vertigo, nausea, sweating, lethargy, headache, flushing Fetal effects: loss of

				variability of fetal heart rate; can cause respiratory depression at birth; can cause decreased muscle tone at birth
Hydroxyzine hydrochloride (Atarax, Vistaril)	Antianxiety agent (minor tranquilizer), antihistamine, antiemetic	IM: 25-50 mg, repeated 4-6 hr prn IM or IV injection	Sedative, antiemetic Duration 3-4 hr	Can reduce amount of narcotic needed Never given by SC, intraarterial
Promethazine hydrochloride (Phenergan)	Antihistaminic, antiemetic	Sedation early labor: 12.5-50 mg Sedation active labor: 25-50 mg with 25-75 mg of meperidine; may be repeated Nausea and vomiting: 12.5-25 mg, repeated 4-6 hr prn	Antihistaminic effects occur within 20 min after IM injection Duration of action 4-6 hr	

ASSESSMENT

A rule of thumb for determining a client's need for analgesia is her inability to relax between contractions. When the client requests pain medication, the nurse assesses her progress in labor and the contraction pattern, as well as the resting tone of the uterus and her vital signs. The FHR is assessed to determine fetal well-being.

FOCUS ASSESSMENT

Determine client's current level of knowledge about the use of analgesia and anesthesia during labor and delivery.

Identify individual client's nonverbal indicators of pain.

Monitor client's behavioral response to uterine contractions.

Determine client's need or desire for analgesia.

Monitor client's physiologic and psychologic response to analgesia, e.g., vital signs, nonverbal indicators of pain, level of consciousness.

Monitor fetal response to analgesia, i.e., heart rate.

Monitor time elapsed between administration of analgesia and signs of impending delivery.

INTERVENTION

NURSING SUPPORT AND COMFORT MEASURES

Position client with pillows and blankets behind her back and between and under her legs to promote relaxation, reduce tension, and eliminate pressure points.

Encourage use of relaxation techniques.

Encourage use of breathing techniques.

Encourage use of effleurage.

Organize procedures to provide for rest.

Control who is present during labor and delivery.

Assure privacy and prevent exposure.

Explain the process and progress of labor.

Keep client clean and dry.

Provide mouth care.

Offer washcloth for wiping face.

Give back rub.

Apply heat or cold to client's lower back.

Suggest client empty her bladder.

Give medication for pain or anxiety.

Provide support during vaginal examinations.

Use physical touch.

Apply heat to lower abdomen.

Control environment to decrease noise.

SELECTION OF ANESTHETIC OR ANALGESIC

The ideal analgesic or anesthetic for labor and delivery would satisfy the following conditions:

It provides satisfactory alleviation of pain for the individual parturient.

It does not interfere significantly with the normal mechanics or progress of labor and delivery.

It is not associated with undue risk to the client.

It is associated with minimum fetal and newborn depression.

It provides safe and satisfactory conditions for the delivery.

It allows early interaction between the mother and her newborn, preferably in the delivery room.

However, no single technique of pain relief fulfills all of the above objectives for every woman.

NURSING CARE PLAN

PAIN MANAGEMENT DURING LABOR

POTENTIAL FOR INJURY (FETAL)—RELATED TO DECREASED PLACENTAL PERFUSION SECONDARY TO EFFECTS OF ANALGESIA OR ANESTHESIA

Goals (expected outcomes)	Interventions	Rationale	Evaluation
Client will maintain adequate placental perfusion as evidenced by the continued absence of signs of fetal distress. Fetal status is unaffected by analgesia.	Encourage maternal use of upright or left or right lateral position during labor.	Enhances placental perfusion; minimizes potential for supine hypotensive syndrome.	Maternal blood pressure remains within normal limits.
	Support effective self-management of labor pain, e.g., effective breathing patterns.	Reduces potential need for analgesia.	FHR consistently remains at 120 to 160.
	Institute immediate actions to counteract effects of maternal hypotension.	Minimizes interruption of blood flow to placenta and fetus.	FHR has absence of late decelerations.
	Turn client on left side or manually displace or support fetus to the maternal left.	Increases placental perfusion.	Compromised fetus responds promptly to interventions; FHR returns to normal range.
	Administer oxygen by face mask at 6 to 8 L/min.	Increases level of oxygen in circulating blood available for maternal and fetal use.	Amniotic fluid is clear with no evidence of meconium caused by hypoxia.

			At birth infant's Apgar score is 8 to 10 at 1 and 5 min.

PAIN—RELATED TO UTERINE CONTRACTIONS AND THE PROCESS OF LABOR

	Notify primary health care provider immediately if actions are unsuccessful.	Enables diagnosis and effective treatment.	
Client will experience effective management of her labor discomfort or pain.	Work through support person.	Reinforces couple's pre-established working relationship.	Couple works effectively together.
	Assist with frequent change of position.	Maintaining one position increases tension and discomfort. Moving allows client a sense of control over some aspect of the experience; promotes comfort; provides distraction.	Client verbalizes that position changes and comfort measures reduce tension and increase comfort.
	Encourage use of upright and left-lateral positions.	Supine position may result in compression of inferior vena cava, causing supine hypotensive syndrome. Left-lateral position enhances placental perfusion.	

Continued

NURSING CARE PLAN

PAIN MANAGEMENT DURING LABOR—continued

Goals (expected outcomes)	Interventions	Rationale	Evaluation
PAIN—RELATED TO UTERINE CONTRACTIONS AND THE PROCESS OF LABOR—cont'd			
	Encourage use of breathing techniques practiced in childbirth education classes. If coach is absent or ineffective, assist with breathing pattern as necessary.	Reinforces previous learning; facilitates and supports application of coping patterns. Assists woman in maintaining control of her behavioral response to pain; enhances and supports coping.	Client verbalizes relief of pain or uses breathing patterns correctly. Client is visibly relaxed throughout and after contractions. Client is coping effectively with labor. FHR indicates good placental perfusion.
	Alert client that contraction is beginning.	Warning signal allows woman to begin use of appropriate breathing/relaxation techniques.	
	Let client know the progress of the contraction, i.e., identify the increment, acme, decrement.	Facilitates short-term coping (one contraction at a time).	

Provide positive reinforcement by complimenting her contraction management.	Supports continuing positive self-image; motivates efforts to maintain control over pain responses.
Provide comfort measures; dry bed, back rubs; perineal care; ice chips, mouth care with lemon and glycerine swabs, wiping face with cool washcloth.	Minimizes annoyance of additional discomforts; allows woman to focus on coping with contractions.
Keep client or couple informed of labor's progress.	Provides psychologic boost, i.e., enhances belief that labor will soon end.
Encourage and assist with relaxation with and between contractions.	Relaxation maximizes uteroplacental perfusion, conserves woman's energy, increases coping abilities, and enhances her comfort.

Continued

NURSING CARE PLAN

PAIN MANAGEMENT DURING LABOR—continued

Goals (expected outcomes)	Interventions	Rationale	Evaluation
PAIN—RELATED TO UTERINE CONTRACTIONS AND THE PROCESS OF LABOR—cont'd			
	Provide client teaching: For clients who have had no previous preparation for childbirth, discuss and demonstrate abdominal and chest breathing; institute other above-described interventions.	Encourages client to focus on breathing rather than on pain. Assists in coping with contraction discomfort or pain; allows woman to control her response to pain.	Client begins using abdominal or chest breathing effectively. Client is visibly more relaxed during contractions. Client relaxes after contraction ends. Client verbalizes increased comfort.
	If woman does not relax between contractions, offer analgesic for pain; answer questions; let client or couple know the decision is theirs. Inform primary health care provider of woman's need or request for aid in cop-	Anxiety and tension increase discomfort and lessen coping ability; lack of relaxation can impede labor progress.	

ing with her contractions and regaining control over her response to pain.

Note and record maternal pulse, respirations, and blood pressure and FHR before administering medication. Administer analgesic as ordered. Note and record maternal and fetal response to analgesic. — Identifies present status and provides baseline for future comparisons.

Ensure immediate availability of narcotic-antagonist medications and resuscitative equipment. — Enables prompt treatment of potential complications caused by narcosis.

Client verbalizes relief of discomfort; visibly regains control over response to labor pain.

Maternal vital signs and FHR remain within normal limits.

INEFFECTIVE INDIVIDUAL COPING—RELATED TO LACK OF KNOWLEDGE ABOUT PROCESS OF LABOR, ANXIETY, FEAR, FATIGUE, INABILITY TO CONTROL OWN RESPONSE TO PAINFUL STIMULI, FEAR OF LOSING CONTROL

Client exhibits successful self-management of the psychologic stress of labor.

Encourage client to deal with contractions one at a time and relax as they end. — Anticipating the next contraction causes tension and discomfort during the rest period; anxiety and

Client is coping effectively with labor.

Continued

Nursing Care Plan

Pain Management During Labor—continued

INEFFECTIVE INDIVIDUAL COPING—RELATED TO LACK OF KNOWLEDGE ABOUT PROCESS OF LABOR, ANXIETY, FEAR, FATIGUE, INABILITY TO CONTROL OWN RESPONSE TO PAINFUL STIMULI, FEAR OF LOSING CONTROL—cont'd

Goals (expected outcomes)	Interventions	Rationale	Evaluation
Client fulfills her expectations for a safe and satisfying childbearing experience.		tension reduce tolerance to pain.	
	Explain sensations that can be expected with progressing labor and procedures.	Reduces anxiety and fear of the unknown.	
	Assist with relaxation and distraction.	Supports coping abilities; relaxation enhances uteroplacental blood flow.	Client is visibly relaxed throughout and after contractions. Client is coping effectively with labor.
	Encourage active participation of support person.	Reduces distress and increases cooperation and comfort; supports established relationship.	The couple works effectively together.

Reinforce effective use of breathing techniques. Provide encouragement and praise.	Supports coping abilities and positive self-image. Communicates understanding of couple's stress and needs and the desire to help.	Client uses breathing patterns correctly. Client or couple actively participates in second stage of labor.
Maintain therapeutic use of self, e.g., tone of voice, touch, nearness.	Maintains rapport and facilitates effective nursing support of the client or couple.	
Institute other measures as described under "Pain" as needed.	Facilitates effective pain management; assists successful coping and satisfactory outcome.	Client expresses satisfaction with labor and delivery management.

FATIGUE—RELATED TO ENERGY EXPENDITURE REQUIRED DURING LABOR, LOSS OF SLEEP, LACK OF FOOD

Client will experience minimum fatigue during labor.	Provide a quiet, restful environment; minimize noise and light as possible.	Encourages relaxation.
	Encourage active participation of support person.	Enhances client's sense of security; supports effective collaboration and coping.

Continued

NURSING CARE PLAN

PAIN MANAGEMENT DURING LABOR—continued

Goals (expected outcomes)	Interventions	Rationale	Evaluation
FATIGUE—RELATED TO ENERGY EXPENDITURE REQUIRED DURING LABOR, LOSS OF SLEEP, LACK OF FOOD—cont'd			
	Reinforce effective breathing techniques.	Assists in coping with contractions.	Client is using breathing techniques effectively.
	Encourage relaxation with and after contractions.	Conserves energy.	Client is responsive to nursing measures, client verbalizes increased comfort and ability to relax.
	Provide comfort measures (e.g., dry bed, back rub, ice chips).	Encourages relaxation.	Client dozes between contractions.
	Offer analgesic if client unable to relax and losing control (see Pain).	Reduces perception of pain, assists relaxation, enables return of control.	

KNOWLEDGE DEFICIT—REGARDING USE OF ANALGESIA FOR LABOR AND DELIVERY

Client will make an informed decision about use of analgesia during her labor.	Explain the actions and anticipated effects of the drug(s).	Identifies the advantages and disadvantages of the specific drug(s).	Client verbalizes understanding of anticipated effects of specific drug on labor and the maternal and fetal status.
	Encourage client or couple to ask questions.	Allows verbalization and exploration of concerns.	
	Explain that the effects will be monitored closely.	Provides reassurance of prompt management of untoward effects.	Client expresses satisfaction with management of pain, labor, and delivery.
	Support (and implement) their decision.	Assures their control over pain management during labor and delivery.	Client or couple self-determines acceptance or refusal of analgesia.

PREGNANCY'S PHYSIOLOGIC IMPLICATIONS FOR ANESTHETIC TECHNIQUES

Pregnancy is associated with an increased sensitivity to most anesthetics, analgesics, and tranquilizers, which makes overdose more likely.

Upper airway edema, normally present in late pregnancy, increases the possibility for airway obstruction.

Changes in pulmonary function and an increased oxygen requirement predispose the parturient to the rapid development of hypoxia, particularly in the second stage of labor or during induction of anesthesia. A 40% increase in pulmonary minute ventilation at term, which may increase further to 300% in the second stage of labor, makes induction of anesthesia with inhalation drugs rapid.

Gastrointestinal tract changes brought about by pregnancy and labor affect many drugs used in labor. Increased nausea and vomiting, prolonged gastric emptying time, and the fact that the maternity client may have recently eaten subject her to an increased risk of pulmonary aspiration of gastric contents with its devastating morbidity and mortality.

Changes in the cardiovascular system, particularly those associated with aortic and vena caval compression by the gravid uterus, predispose the obstetric client to sudden hypotension and cardiovascular collapse and her fetus to hypoxia and acidosis at the time of general or major conduction anesthesia.

FORMS OF REGIONAL ANESTHESIA

Subarachnoid block
   Spinal
   Saddle
Peridural (epidural) block
   Lumbar epidural
   Caudal epidural
Paracervical block
Pudendal block
Local infiltration

EFFECTS OF SELECTED REGIONAL ANALGESIC OR ANESTHETIC METHODS AND AGENTS

Types of regional analgesia/anesthesia	Therapeutic effect	Maternal side effects	Fetal or newborn side effects	Miscellaneous information
Subarachnoid block: spinal and saddle	High degree of pain relief for delivery	Maternal hypotension Occasional postspinal headache Urinary retention post partum	None unless maternal hypotension occurs	No pain relief during first stage of labor Excellent pain relief for delivery
Peridural (epidural) block: lumbar and caudal	High degree of pain relief for first and second stage labor and delivery	Frequent mild hypotension; loss of bearing-down reflex in second stage	None unless severe sustained maternal hypotension occurs	May slow labor Epidural blocks pain at each stage of labor Incorrect placement of caudal needle could result in puncture of maternal rectum or fetal head

Continued

EFFECTS OF SELECTED REGIONAL ANALGESIC OR ANESTHETIC METHODS AND AGENTS—continued

Types of regional analgesia/anesthesia	Therapeutic effect	Maternal side effects	Fetal or newborn side effects	Miscellaneous information
Paracervical block	Temporary block of pain during labor	Transient depression of contractions Rare maternal side effects	Fairly high incidence of bradycardia of 25%-85% Contraindications: Premature fetus Fetal compromise Placental insufficiency Vaginal infection	Provides analgesia during labor but no perineal anesthesia; does not interfere with pushing
Pudendal block	Nerve block for second stage of labor	Loss of bearing-down reflex	Rarely any	Does not relieve contraction pain; anesthetizes perineum

REGIONAL ANALGESIC AND ANESTHETIC AGENTS

Local anesthetic and trade name	Characteristics	Route	Comments
Chloroprocaine (Nesacaine)	Very low toxicity, most rapidly metabolized anesthetic, with little accumulation and rapid onset but poor spread; short duration of action	Caudal, epidural, spinal, pudendal	Ideal drug for epidural; rapid onset, rapid rate of hydrolysis; low fetal or maternal toxicity
Tetracaine (Pontocaine)	Poor spread, very slow onset	Spinal (subarachnoid block)	Only made for spinal block (too toxic for epidural or caudal)
Lidocaine (Xylocaine)	Most versatile local anesthetic, moderate toxicity, rapid onset, moderate duration, excellent spread	Caudal, epidural, spinal, pudendal, and paracervical block	With epidural use, possible suppression of some reflexes in newborn; recent studies question this conclusion
Mepivacaine (Carbocaine)	Rapid onset, moderate duration, moderate toxicity but very slow metabolism, marked accumulation with repeated dosage	Caudal, epidural, spinal, paracervical block, pudendal	Epidural use associated with minimum decrease in temporary neonatal muscle tone

Continued

REGIONAL ANALGESIC AND ANESTHETIC AGENTS—continued

Local anesthetic and trade name	Characteristics	Route	Comments
Bupivacaine (Marcaine, Sensorcaine)	Slow onset, long duration, marked cardiac toxicity; low concentrations give excellent sensory and little motor block, ideal for obstetrics	Caudal, epidural, paracervical block, pudendal	Inadvertent intravascular injection associated with cardiovascular collapse
Etidocaine (Duranest)	Rapid onset, long duration, marked cardiac toxicity; produces profound motor block and often poor sensory block, making it a poor drug for obstetrics	Caudal, epidural, paracervical block, pudendal	Inadvertent intravascular injection associated with cardiovascular collapse

Chapter 5

FIRST STAGE OF LABOR

This chapter presents the three phases of the first stage of labor. The nurse's role is one of support person for the mother and coach and to maintain the well-being of the mother and fetus during this initial stage.

ASSESSMENT

CHARACTERISTICS OF UTERINE CONTRACTIONS IN FIRST STAGE OF LABOR

	Latent phase of labor	Active phase of labor	Transition phase of labor
Frequency	5 min	3-3½ min	2-2½ min
Duration	30-50 sec	60-75 sec	60-90 sec
Intensity			
Internal monitor	25-40 mm Hg Intrauterine Pressure	40-60 mm Hg Intrauterine Pressure	60-75 mm Hg Intrauterine Pressure
External monitor: palpation of contraction at peak by nurse	Fundus dents at peak	Fundus firm at peak difficult to indent	Fundus very firm or hard at peak
Uterine tonus			
Internal monitor	Average 8-12 mm Hg	Same	Same
	No greater than 15-20 mm Hg	Same	Same
External monitor: palpation by nurse between contractions	Relaxed	Same	Same
Shape of contractions	Bell-shaped	Bell-shaped	Bell-shaped

DEVIATIONS FROM EXPECTED PATTERNS: CONTRACTION WARNING SIGNS

1. Hypertonus: relaxation between contractions not adequate; if IUP in place, resting tone is greater than 20 mm Hg.
2. Relaxation phase between contractions less than 60 seconds.
3. Contractions greater than 90 seconds in duration.
4. Contractions exceeding 90 mm Hg in intensity.

ADMISSION HISTORY AND NURSING ASSESSMENT

1. Date and time of admission
2. Primary care provider (obstetrician, family practice physician, or certified nurse midwife)
3. Infant's physician or pediatrician
4. Estimated date of confinement (delivery)—note if determined by dates or by ultrasound
5. Gravida, para, abortions
6. Allergies
7. Maternal medical-surgical history (i.e., heart disease, diabetes, high blood pressure, any other problems)
8. Medications or drugs taken during pregnancy
9. Any problems with previous pregnancies
10. Any problems with this pregnancy
11. When labor began, when contractions became 5 min apart and regular (primigravida) as 5 to 10 min and regular (multipara)
12. Contractions on admission: frequency, duration, frequency, relaxation
13. Vaginal discharge
    a. Membranes intact or ruptured? Date, time, amount, appearance, color, and odor if ruptured
    b. Bloody show or frank bleeding? Type, amount, color (include when it began)
14. Last oral intake: what and when
15. Vital signs: temperature, pulse, respirations, blood pressure
16. Fetal heart rate: rate, location, regularity
17. Vaginal examination findings: dilatation, effacement, presentation, and station
18. Labor plans discussed with primary care provider

Sample Narrative Charting: ADMISSION NOTE—Primigravida admitted to Labor, Delivery, Recovery Room (LDR) No. 5 in labor. Changed clothes and into bed. Oriented to surroundings. Contractions 3-3½ minutes apart, lasting 60 seconds, and good quality. States "contractions hurt." Husband present and coaching through contractions. Working well together. BP 110/60 (between contractions on left side). TPR 98.6-84-18. Vaginal exam done. External fetal monitor applied, hooked into central station. Oriented to monitor. Signal cord within reach. Dr. Edmiston notified of admission and assessment.

INITIAL FETAL ASSESSMENT

1. Is the fetus mature? What is the due date?
2. Are the client's membranes ruptured? If so, what is the color of the amniotic fluid (clear, meconium stained)? Consistency of fluid (thick, thin)? Odor? Any bloody show or bleeding?
3. Does the mother look as though she is carrying a term fetus? Measure fundal height and correlate with gestational age.
4. Is the fetus active? Has the mother noticed any changes or decrease in fetal movement?
5. Auscultate the fetal heart for baseline rate and rhythm, or apply the electronic fetal monitor and run a strip of tracing to assess baseline FHR, reactivity, and any periodic changes.

FETAL HEART RATE (FHR)

Finding	Beats per minute (bpm)
Normal baseline range at term*	120-160
Mild tachycardia	160-180
Marked tachycardia	>180
Mild bradycardia	100-119
Marked bradycardia	<100

*Baseline FHR is the rate between contractions (or when the client is not in labor).

INTERVENTION

APPLICATION OF EXTERNAL FETAL MONITOR

Intervention

1. Explain procedure to mother (and coach).
2. Lay out transducer (to monitor the contraction pattern) and tocodynamometer (toco).
3. Place both monitor belts beneath mother's back.
4. Plug transducer and toco into monitor and press button for power.
5. Place toco on mother's abdomen at level of her umbilicus. Secure toco according to manufacturer's guidelines so that contractions can be recorded. Note: Toco only records frequency, duration and shape of contractions.
6. Apply ultrasonic gel to underneath side of transducer.
7. Place transducer on area of abdomen identified as appropriate for receiving best fetal heart signal.

Rationale

1. Helps to dispel anxiety and fear
2. Orients couple to monitor and its attachments.
3. For securing transducer and toco after placement in appropriate area on abdomen
4. All equipment now ready to function
5. If toco placed above umbilicus, monitors mother's respiratory rate instead of FHR.

6. Aids in transmission of sound waves
7. Initial transducer placement; some adjustment may be needed

APPLICATION OF EXTERNAL FETAL MONITOR—continued

Intervention

8. Increase volume and listen for FHR. If signal not optimum, readjust transducer placement (wait 3-4 sec between moves of transducer).

9. When placement of monitor is complete, document the following:
   a. Application of external monitor
   b. Date and time of application
   c. Average baseline FHR
   d. Monitor connected to central bank (some hospitals have displays at nurses' station (or other locations) that receive the most recent 7-8 min of fetal heart and contraction tracings from each client's room)

Rationale

8. Locates best site for receiving fetal heart signal; 3-4 sec pause between adjusting permits monitor to develop its memory of information received

9. Documentation necessary for every procedure

NURSING CARE PLAN

FIRST STAGE OF LABOR

INEFFECTIVE INDIVIDUAL OR FAMILY COPING—RELATED TO HOSPITALIZATION OR CLIENT'S BEING IN PAIN

Goals (expected outcomes)	Interventions	Rationale	Evaluation
Client and her support person benefit from having worked together as a team throughout the first stage of labor.	Encourage support person's participation in care.	Promotes effective coping by binding client and support person closer.	Support person assists client in coping with labor.
	Work through support person for change of position or change in breathing.	Helps support person feel needed and good about involvement.	Support person states he or she feels part of the labor process.
	Provide explanations to client and support person.	Assists support person in helping the client.	Client states she benefits from support person's presence and support.
	Identify and reinforce adaptive coping behavior.	Makes support person aware of importance of job and that job is being well done (essential part of the team).	Support person feels that he or she is doing a good job.
	Provide support to support person (refreshments and breaks).	Promotes support person's ability to cope since he or she also needs refreshments and breaks but often feels guilty about leaving unless suggestion comes from nurse.	Support person expresses gratitude that breaks are suggested.

FEAR—RELATED TO HOSPITAL PROCEDURES AND SURROUNDINGS AND LABOR (AND IMPENDING DELIVERY)

Client reports increased comfort with hospital procedures and process of labor and delivery.	Provide calm, quiet environment.	Assists client to be calm.	Client is relaxed, showing no anxiety and fear.
	Anticipate unasked questions and give explanation for everything to be done.	Eliminates fear of unknown.	Client appears more confident about progress.
	Give positive feedback for progress.	Increases her confidence in herself, reducing anxiety.	Client states she is grateful for praise.
	Reinforce that client and baby are both doing well if realistic (i.e., all vital signs of both are normal).	Accentuates the positive, gives mother more confidence that she and her infant are doing OK. Promotes positive feelings.	Client verbalizes she is more confident and less fearful.

ALTERATION IN TISSUE PERFUSION—RELATED TO SUPINE POSITION CAUSING COMPRESSION OF INFERIOR VENA CAVA AND AORTA AND DECREASED PLACENTAL PERFUSION TO FETUS

Client and fetus progress through first stage of labor with no problems.	Maintain position of client in lateral or upright position.	Prevents compression of vena cava and aorta by uterus and fetus.	Client remains normotensive and voices no complaints of nausea or dizziness.

Continued

Nursing Care Plan

First Stage of Labor—continued

Goals (expected outcomes)	Interventions	Rationale	Evaluation
ALTERATION IN TISSUE PERFUSION—RELATED TO SUPINE POSITION CAUSING COMPRESSION OF INFERIOR VENA CAVA AND AORTA AND DECREASED PLACENTAL PERFUSION TO FETUS—cont'd			
	Place wedge under client's right hip for vaginal examinations, induction of epidural anesthesia, and any other procedures requiring a supine position.	Offsets uterus and fetus from the inferior vena cava and aorta.	Fetus maintains normal baseline rate (absence of tachycardia, bradycardia or late decelerations).
	Place wedge under client's right hip if supine position necessary.	Keeps uterus and fetus off aorta and vena cava.	Blood pressure and FHR remain stable.
ACUTE PAIN—RELATED TO PROGRESS OF LABOR			
Client demonstrates an understanding of how to help and par-	Change position every one-half hour (side lying and upright).	Promotes comfort and maintains contraction pattern.	Client appears relaxed between contractions and has stable contraction pattern.

ticipate, to maximize her comfort, and to help determine if and when analgesia will be used.

Interventions	Rationale	Outcomes
Permit ambulation until membranes rupture and presenting part engaged.	Promotes comfort and facilitates contractions and progress in labor.	Client has regular stable contraction pattern and states pain is tolerable.
Encourage relaxation and distraction.	Passes time, decreases discomfort, facilitates progress of labor.	Client is relaxed and participates in making decisions about position changes and use of analgesia.
Promote effective breathing techniques as long as they are helpful.	Aids coping with contractions.	Couple works together well with breathing and relaxation.
Encourage use of visual imagery.	Provides distraction.	Client verbalizes coping success with contractions.
Provide warm shower or bath if physician agrees (if bag of water intact).	Promotes relaxation and progress.	Client states she is relaxed and feels good about coping skills.
Assist with comfort measures: giving back rub, performing effleurage, wiping face, keeping bed straightened and dry, maintaining comfortable room temperature, giving perineum care as needed.	Aids in promoting comfort.	Client states all comfort measures are helpful and facilitate effective coping.

Continued

NURSING CARE PLAN

FIRST STAGE OF LABOR—continued

Goals (expected outcomes)	Interventions	Rationale	Evaluation
ACUTE PAIN—RELATED TO PROGRESS OF LABOR—cont'd			
	Promote privacy and quiet environment.	Promotes comfort.	Client appears relaxed and verbalizes that environment is restful.
	Assist with regulation of visitors.	May need assistance in regulating who stays and who leaves.	Client verbalizes positive responses to limiting visitors.
	Provide clear fluids or ice chips.	Provides oral hygiene and hydration.	Client states mouth does not feel dry at present.
	Administer intravenous fluids as ordered; observe for bladder distention.	Provides hydration.	Client is able to void approximately every 2 hr.
	Encourage voiding every 1-3 hr.	Full bladder may impede descent of fetus.	Client's bladder is empty, and fetus is descending.
	Provide encouragement to mother and her support person.	Both need reassurance they are doing well.	Client and support person verbalize pleasure at a job well done.
	Administer analgesic as	Assists with pain management	Client is coping well and is

	more relaxed after receiving analgesic. FHR pattern is normal.
and relaxation to facilitate fetal oxygenation.	
ordered when mother unable to relax between contractions.	

KNOWLEDGE DEFICIT—REGARDING PROCESS OF LABOR AND HOSPITAL PROCEDURES AND ROUTINE

Goal	Intervention	Rationale	Expected Outcome
Childbirth plans are fulfilled and satisfied.	Explain what sensations to expect in each phase of first stage of labor, e.g., contraction pattern will increase.	Assists understanding of each phase of labor and why contractions are more frequent, last longer, and are more intense.	Client verbalizes and demonstrates understanding of labor, hospital procedures, and routine.
	Explain procedures to be done, what to expect, and reason for each.	Prepares for what is to be done and why it is done.	Client verbalizes understanding of procedures; states it is easier when she knows what to expect.
	Encourage questions; clarify and explain as needed.	Provides optimum atmosphere for providing information.	Client asks questions to clarify understanding.
	Explain need to call for nurse if bag of water ruptures.	Assures client knows why calling for nurse is important.	Client calls for nurse when membranes rupture.
	Explain need for ambulation (if indicated), position changes, emptying of bladder, relaxation.	Increases knowledge and positive working with the labor.	Client initiates changes in position and is cooperative.
	Reinforce good work that both are doing.	Causes them to try even harder.	Both respond to praise and work harder to do well.

Continued

Nursing Care Plan

ADMISSION OF CLIENT IN LABOR

Goals (expected outcomes)	Interventions	Rationale	Evaluation
ACUTE PAIN—RELATED TO UTERINE CONTRACTIONS AND CERVICAL DILATATION			
Client will experience effective management of pain during labor and delivery.	Assess client's response to pain; give encouragement to couple. Assist with pain-relief techniques.	Determines effectiveness of coping and ensures couple is given help to experience what they desire from this childbearing experience.	Client reports satisfaction with the pain control experienced during labor.
	Encourage and support client's participation in choice of technique to cope with pain.	Both client and coach need to feel they are in control and doing a good job.	Client verbalizes satisfaction with labor experience and support of nurse.
	Encourage relationships by providing quiet, restful environment, keeping client clean and dry, and monitoring breathing techniques.	Helps in coping with labor pain.	Client appears relaxed during contractions.
	During contractions assist coach to give sacral pressure for backache.	Counter pressure to sacrum often decreases severity of backache.	Client reports that severity of backache decreases with sacral massage.

Encourage client to ambulate if permitted.	Decreases pain perception.	Client reports contractions are less painful while ambulating.
Offer ice chips, lip balm.	Prevents dry mouth and cracked lips; may help decrease thirst.	Client reports that ice chips decrease thirst.
Support client in choice of analgesia or anesthesia.	Client makes informed choice to meet her pain needs.	Client expresses choice of analgesia or anesthesia.

ALTERED PLACENTAL PERFUSION TO FETUS—RELATED TO MOTHER'S SUPINE POSITION

Client will maintain sidelying or upright position.	Teach importance of never lying in supine position.	Minimizes potential for supine hypotension; maximizes venous return of blood to heart and maximizes cardiac output.	Client avoids supine position, displays no signs of hypotension; FHR baseline is stable.

INEFFECTIVE INDIVIDUAL COPING—RELATED TO LACK OF SUPPORT SYSTEMS

Client will cope effectively with contractions.	Encourage presence of support person(s). Nurse will assist with support if no support person is available. Assist support person in coaching breathing techniques.	Studies have shown that mothers and fetuses do better if support person is present.	Client maintained appropriate breathing patterns. Relaxes between contractions.

Continued

Nursing Care Plan

Admission of Client in Labor—continued

Goals (expected outcomes)	Interventions	Rationale	Evaluation

INEFFECTIVE INDIVIDUAL COPING—RELATED TO LACK OF SUPPORT SYSTEMS—cont'd

Interventions:

Make sure support person gets breaks.

Praise support person.

Talk to mother and support person as a team, giving encouragement and praise.

Instruct support person.

Wipe mother's face with cool wash cloth.

Offer ice chips.

Tell mother when contraction begins and when it is ending.

Rub mother's back.

Instruct support person about how to determine if mother is relaxing.

KNOWLEDGE DEFICIT—REGARDING PROCESS OF LABOR AND BODY CHANGES

Client will gain understanding of what is happening to her and what to expect.	Establish relationship with client and support person.	Provides reassurance, care and effective communication.	Client and support person are familiar with the new environment and "settle in."
	Learn how clients want to be addressed (e.g., first name).	Increases psychological comfort.	Client states how she wants to be addressed.
	Provide orientation to the unit and labor process.	Decreases tension or anxiety related to the "unknown".	Client understands equipment, procedures, expectations.
	Convey attitude that the couple is expected and welcomed.	Provides warm, comfortable, and therapeutic atmosphere.	Client states she is comfortable with the environment and the nurse.
	Individualize teaching plan to cover expectations and restrictions of the environment; review or teach relaxation methods and answer questions.	Personalizes the labor experience.	Client and support person(s) state they feel rapport with the nurse(s).
	Explain the fetal monitor and how it works.	Provides confidence and eliminates fear of technology.	Client states she feels reassured by hearing the infant's heart beat.

Chapter 6

SECOND STAGE OF LABOR

The second stage of labor begins with complete dilatation of the cervix and ends with delivery of the baby. The usual duration of second stage is approximately 1 hour for the primigravida and one-half hour for the multipara.

ASSESSMENT

SIGNS AND SYMPTOMS INDICATING ONSET OF SECOND STAGE OF LABOR

- Involuntary bearing down caused by the Ferguson reflex when the presenting part is near or on the perineal floor.
- Sudden increase in bloody show caused by exposure of cervical capillaries as a result of increasing cervical dilatation (and effacement).
- Rupture of membranes, which may occur at any time but occurs frequently at the beginning of the second stage.
- Urge to defecate, caused by pressure of the presenting part against the rectum.
- Bulging of perineum and dilatation of anal orifice.
- Increased apprehension and irritability or relief and elation at being able to push to shorten time of delivery.

CHARACTERISTICS OF UTERINE CONTRACTIONS DURING SECOND STAGE

Frequency	Duration	Intensity	Uterine Tonus	Shape of Contractions
3-3½ min	60-75 sec	Internal monitor: 40-60 mm Hg intrauterine pressure External monitor: palpation of contraction at peak by nurse—fundus firm; client pushing with contractions	Internal monitor: average 8-12 mm Hg; >15-20 mm Hg is hypertonus External monitor: fundus palpation by nurse between contractions to ensure it is relaxed	Bell shaped

PERIODIC FETAL HEART RATE CHANGES

Accelerations: Caused by umbilical vein compression
Early decelerations: Caused by fetal head compression
Late decelerations: Caused by uteroplacental insufficiency
Variable decelerations: Caused by complete cord compression

CLINICAL SIGNIFICANCE OF THE FETAL HEART RATE

Baseline Fetal Heart Rate (FHR)
Definition: the average FHR when woman is *not* in labor; the average FHR *between* labor contractions (10 min of tracing must be assessed to determine baseline)
Normal FHR: 120-160 beats/min
Tachycardia: >160 beats/min; associated with the following:
    Maternal fever
    Chronic fetal hypoxia

Fetal immaturity

Maternal anemia

Administration of betamimetic drugs for inhibition of preterm labor

Intrauterine sepsis

Stress and/or anxiety

Bradycardia: <120 beats/min (more real concern when <100 beats/min; associated with the following:

Significant interruption of the blood flow carrying O_2 to fetus

Late fetal hypoxia (terminal event)

Congenital heart lesions

Maternal hypotension

Postdatism

Periodic Change in FHR

Definition: FHR change during the contraction

Early deceleration: begins, peaks, and goes away with contraction shape; associated with the following:

Increased pressure on head

Late deceleration: uniform; begins at the peak or after the acme of the contraction; associated with the following:

Decreased maternal-fetal O_2 exchange

Decreased utero-placental insufficiency

Maternal hypoxia

Maternal position (supine), causing compression of inferior vena cava and aorta (may cause maternal hypotension)

Uterine hyperactivity

Variable deceleration: occurs at any point in the contraction (most common periodic change FHR—an important periodic fetal heart pattern); associated with the following:

Umbilical cord compression

FHR Variability

Definition: beat-to-beat changes in FHR that vary from the baseline

Short term: beat-to-beat changes occurring within a few heartbeats

Long term: gradual changes in the interval length (range of the FHR over 10 minutes)

Note: Variability has become the most important aspect of the overall clinical evaluation of the fetus in utero.

INTERVENTION

INTRAUTERINE RESUSCITATION

Intervention

1. Change position of mother.

2. Turn off oxytocin if running.

3. Hydrate; begin intravenous infusion or increase rate so approximately 200 ml/15 min will infuse.

4. Administer 6-8 L oxygen through snug face mask.

5. If mother is pushing, encourage her to discontinue pushing until FHR improves.

6. Stimulate the fetus; stimulate scalp or use vibroaccoustic stimulator.

7. If hyperstimulation continues, notify primary care provider.

8. Be prepared to assist with scalp sampling if none of above interventions are effective.

9. Notify primary care provider of all interventions and their effects on the fetal heart.

10. Document interventions on tracing as they are done and summarize in nurses' notes in a timely fashion.

Rationale

1. Relieves pressure on compressed inferior vena cava and aorta and relieves pressure on compressed umbilical cord.

2. Decreased uterine activity may increase uteroplacental circulation.

3. Increases maternal circulatory volume so blood and oxygen are optimally perfusing uterus and placenta.

4. Increases oxygen flow to uterus and placenta.

5. After tracing improved, titrate pushing with FHR reading to ensure best oxygenation.

6. If acceleration occurs, fetus is not decompensated (acidotic); if no acceleration occurs, use chain of command to get physician.

7. Anticipate an order for terbutaline sulfate (Brethine), 0.25 ml.

8. Determines whether acidosis is present based on pH of scalp blood sample.

9. Prepares for emergency delivery or cesarean section.

10. Provides accurate current record of occurrences and interventions.

CLIENT SELF-CARE EDUCATION

PUSHING DURING SECOND STAGE OF LABOR

Intervention

1. Examine client to determine if cervix is completely dilated.
2. Assist her to achieve position of comfort—more upright (or lateral recumbent).
3. Encourage coach to tell client when a contraction is beginning.
4. Instruct client to take two or three cleansing breaths until contraction intensity increases.
5. Instruct client to push spontaneously for no longer than 6 sec while emitting grunting or moaning sounds.
6. Instruct client to rest briefly between pushing efforts (usually takes three breaths or has 2 sec between pushes).
7. Support client's voluntary pushing efforts.
8. Assess client for vulvar bulging and for crowning.

Rationale

1. Pushing should not begin before dilatation is complete.
2. Upright position facilitates descent.
3. Prepares client for beginning of contraction.
4. Pushing is more effective nearer acme of contraction.
5. Gives control to client and negates Valsalva maneuver.
6. Minimizes fall of oxygen tension (Po_2) and rise of carbon dioxide tension (Pco_2).
7. Labor may last longer but also results in fetal, neonatal, and maternal well-being.
8. Indicates imminence of delivery.

NURSING CARE PLAN

SECOND STAGE OF LABOR

Goals (expected outcomes)	Interventions	Rationale	Evaluation
INEFFECTIVE INDIVIDUAL COPING—RELATED TO PHYSICAL EXHAUSTION IN RESPONSE TO LABOR			
Client will proceed through second stage of labor with minimum exhaustion and will feel she has done a good job.	Promote relaxation and rest between contractions. Provide quiet environment.	Conserves strength and decreases exhaustion. Promotes maximum rest.	Client is rested and relaxed between contractions. Same as above.
	Encourage active participation of support system.	Enhances their working effectiveness and team effort.	Client and support person state they feel good about their team effort.
	Praise client's pushing efforts.	Promotes continued pushing efforts.	Client verbalizes positions she prefers for pushing.
	Praise support person for doing good coaching.	Increases feelings of worth and helping.	
	Suggest alternative positions for pushing (upright, squatting, knee chest, lateral recumbent).	Increases alignment of fetus to pelvis; uses forces of gravity.	Client states she has increased urge to push; pushing feels more effective.
	Assist in promoting constructive behaviors.	Helps client feel positive about her role (clients need firm, but kind coaching).	Client is pleased with her behavior during labor.

Continued

NURSING CARE PLAN

SECOND STAGE OF LABOR—continued

Goals (expected outcomes)	Interventions	Rationale	Evaluation
PAIN—RELATED TO INCREASING INTENSITY OF CONTRACTIONS			
Client will understand the alterations available for pain control and make decisions to manage her pain or discomfort.	Assess response to pain; give encouragement and suggestions to help cope.	Accents the positive and helps client cope.	Client appears in control and uses suggestions.
	Review tools that provide most help to client: deep ventilation before and after contraction; use of breathing technique and pushing with contractions; short pushes rather than sustained ones; relaxation between contractions.	Assists client's remembering the tools (using familiar tools may be helpful).	Client uses tools that help the most.
	Continue coaching to push.	Increases descent.	Fetus is descending 1 cm/hr primigravida, 2 cm/hr multipara.

	Monitor maternal and fetal vital signs with every contraction during push and after contraction.	More potential for problems as labor progresses.	Client has normal vital signs; fetus has normal baseline FHR and no decelerations.
	Assist with positioning for induction of anesthesia.	Difficult to curl around baby with close, hard contractions.	Anesthesia was given with no difficulty.
	Continue helping to coach during pushing.	Ensures client and fetus are OK.	Client's vital signs are normal; fetus has normal baseline FHR and no decelerations.

ALTERATION IN PERFUSION (UTERO-PLACENTAL-FETAL)—RELATED TO INCREASED FREQUENCY, DURATION, INTENSITY OF CONTRACTIONS

Client and fetus will progress through second stage without problems.	Maintain client's upright, or side-lying position.	Maximizes utero-placental fetal blood flow and assists with normal contraction pattern.	Client maintains appropriate positions.
	Coach pushing efforts: no closed glottis pushing; no push greater than 6 sec.	Maintains normal maternal acid-base balance.	Client and fetus are well oxygenated.
	Assess maternal vital signs and FHR.	Assesses maternal and fetal well-being and recognizes if problems occur.	Client's vital signs are normal; fetus has reassuring FHR pattern.

Continued

NURSING CARE PLAN

SECOND STAGE OF LABOR—continued

Goals (expected outcomes)	Interventions	Rationale	Evaluation
ALTERATION IN PERFUSION (UTERO-PLACENTAL-FETAL)—RELATED TO INCREASED FREQUENCY, DURATION, INTENSITY OF CONTRACTIONS—cont'd			
	Record on strip and chart every intervention, client's response, presence or absence of pain, fetal responses.	Provides legal record of nursing assessment and interventions.	All documentation is complete and up-to-date.
FEAR—RELATED TO SECOND STAGE OF LABOR AND IMMINENT DELIVERY OF THE FETUS			
Couple will fulfill birth plan through constant support for and confidence in their abilities.	Explain what is happening as it happens.	Helps dispel fear and increases understanding; promotes compliance.	Couple verbalizes understanding of pushing and delivery and appears more relaxed.

Continuously encourage and reinforce couple's efforts and coping strategies and keep them informed of progress.	Perpetuates the positive efforts; gives positive strokes.	Couple participates, is effectively compliant, and is pleased with their experience.
Provide environment conducive to couple's work. Ask what will make environment more comfortable.	Enables couple to work and cope their best.	Couple participates effectively.
Encourage client to push according to perceived urge; add tips that will enhance the pushing.	Allows mother to push when it feels most effective and natural for her to do so; nurse's tips assist.	Fetus descends progressively.
Notify anesthesiologist and primary care giver when delivery is imminent.	Ensures appropriate medical assistance available for delivery.	Delivery occurs with no problems.
Prepare for delivery.	Ensures enough time for setting up so that everything needed is available and working.	All delivery equipment is prepared in time for safe, expeditious delivery.

Chapter 7

OPERATIVE OBSTETRICS

There are several special procedures the physician may use to assist the mother in labor and delivery. These include induction of labor, use of forceps, laceration repair, and cesarean birth.

SOME INDICATIONS AND CONTRAINDICATIONS FOR INDUCTION OF LABOR

Indications	Contraindications
Pregnancy-induced hypertension	Placenta previa
Premature rupture of membranes	Abnormal fetal presentation
Choriamnionitis	Cord presentation
Suspected fetal jeopardy as evidenced by biochemical or biophysical indications, e.g., fetal growth retardation, postterm gestation, isoimmunization	Presenting part above the pelvic inlet
	Prior classic uterine incision
	Active genital herpes infection
	Pelvic structural deformities
	Invasive cervical carcinoma
Maternal medical problems, e.g., diabetes mellitus, renal disease, chronic obstructive pulmonary disease	
Fetal demise	
Logistic factors, e.g., risk of rapid labor, distance from hospital	
Postterm gestation	

From NAACOG: The nurse's role in induction/augmentation of labor. OGN Nurs Pract Resource, January 1988.

OXYTOCIN ADMINISTRATION

TIPS ABOUT CONTRACTIONS (WITH OR WITHOUT USE OF OXYTOCIN)

There is a relationship between *frequency* of contractions and *intensity* of contractions.

As contraction *frequency* increases, contraction *intensity* decreases.

OR

As contraction *intensity* increases, contraction *frequency* decreases.

PHARMACOLOGIC RESPONSE OF UTERUS TO OXYTOCIN

Incremental phase—as oxytocin is increased, uterine activity increases.

Stable phase—uterine activity continues to increase until a stable phase of contractions is established, i.e., frequency, duration, quality, shape, and resting tone. Contraction pattern no longer requires stimulation with oxytocin.

If oxytocin is increased, contractions become too frequent and resting tone of uterus will increase, resulting in tetany.

ASSESSMENT

OXYTOCIN INFUSION: SIGNS OF HYPERSTIMULATION OF THE UTERUS

Maternal
1. Contractions occur more frequently than every 2 minutes.
2. Duration of contraction is longer than 90 seconds.
3. Elevation of resting tone of uterus (hypertonus) is greater than 15 to 20 mm Hg by intrauterine pressure catheter. Uterine palpation reveals loss of complete relaxation between contractions.
4. Blood pressure increases when contractions increase in frequency, duration, and intensity because of decrease in uteroplacental circulation.
5. Client experiences increasing pain because of increased frequency, duration, and intensity of contractions.
6. Sustained tetanic contractions occur.

Fetal
1. Tachycardia or bradycardia.
2. Late decelerations, variable decelerations, or prolonged deceleration.
3. Loss of variability.
4. Increased fetal activity due to decreased oxygenation.

Sample Narrative Charting: Contractions are 1½ to 4½ minutes apart, duration 40 to 45 seconds, intensity 50 to 70 mm Hg, and resting tone is 5 to 15 mm Hg. Baseline FHR 155. Decreased long- and short-term variability. Repetitive late decelerations are occurring. Positioned on left side. Pitocin discontinued. Mainline infusion increased. Oxygen started at 8 L/min by face mask. Cervix is 5 to 6 cm, 90% effaced, station is 0. Moderate amount of fresh bloody show. Leaking meconium-stained fluid. Relaxing well between contractions. Husband helping with breathing during contractions. Explained interventions initiated and that physician is coming in to assess situation. Concerned but state they are glad physician is coming.

INTERVENTION

PREPARING AND ADMINISTERING OXYTOCIN INFUSION

Intervention	Rationale
1. Explain procedure and rationale to client.	1. An informed client is less anxious and fearful.
2. Apply fetal monitor and monitor the FHR to establish a baseline tracing.	2. Ensures fetal reactivity.
3. Start an electrolytes solution IV infusion, called the primary line.	3. An electrolyte solution minimizes the risk of water intoxication.
4. Prepare a second IV (secondary line) and add the prescribed amount of oxytocin (usually 10 U/1000 ml). The IV tubing is inserted into the infusion controller (or pump) and primed to clear air from the line.	4. Oxytocin must be administered with an infusion pump (or controller) to ensure accurate dose administration.
5. "Piggyback" the secondary line into the primary line at the port closest to the needle insertion site and then turn on at the prescribed rate of infusion.	5. The secondary line contains the oxytocin. If there is an indication to stop the oxytocin infusion, it can be done without affecting the infusion of the primary line, and fluid volume can be maintained.

Adapted from NAACOG: The nurse's role in the induction/augmentation of labor. OGN Nurs Pract Resource, January 1988.

PREPARING AND ADMINISTERING OXYTOCIN INFUSION— continued

Intervention	Rationale
6. Turn on oxytocin infusion pump at prescribed rate.	6. No other medications should be given through the oxytocin (secondary) line, since it will be given at prescribed rates and may be turned off if contractions are too close, hypertonus occurs, or the FHR pattern indicates fetal distress.
7. Monitor FHR, uterine resting tone, frequency, duration and intensity of contractions, blood pressure, and pulse and record at intervals comparable to the *dosage regimen,* i.e., at 30- to 60-minute intervals, when the dosage is evaluated for maintenance, increase, or decrease. Evidence of maternal and fetal surveillance should be documented. All observations and increases or decreases in oxytocin are documented on the fetal heart tracing and the mother's chart.	7. If uterus becomes hyperstimulated, blood flow to uteroplacental site will be decreased and fetus will suffer from hypoxia.
8. Once the desired frequency of contractions has been reached and labor has progressed to 5 to 6 cm dilatation, oxytocin may be reduced by similar increments (or as prescribed by physician).	8. Sensitivity to oxytocin increases as labor progresses. If stable pattern is achieved, need for oxytocin decreases.

Continued

PREPARING AND ADMINISTERING OXYTOCIN INFUSION— continued

Intervention

9. If hyperstimulation of the uterus occurs (less than 2 minutes between contractions and lasting longer than 60 seconds) or a nonreassuring fetal heart rate pattern occurs, the following actions are taken:
   a. Turn off oxytocin infusion
   b. Speed up primary infusion
   c. Change position, may turn to left side
   d. Give oxygen 6 to 8 min by face mask
   e. Notify charge nurse (supervisor) and physician STAT
   f. Provide support to parents
   g. Document on monitor strip and client's chart
   h. Document effectiveness of interventions

10. Notify the physician of hypertonic/hypotonic contractions or failure to progress.

11. Continue to assess client's progress, both physically and emotionally (care is for the client, not the monitor).

Rationale

9. Intrauterine resuscitation is initiated when there is significant interruption of oxygenation due to decrease or cessation of utero-placental perfusion.

10. Clients may vary in their individual responsiveness to oxytocin. Some may require more; some less.

11. Induced or augmented labor is stressful to couple. The nurse is attuned to their responses and intervenes as indicated. They need to know that progress is occurring.

PREPARING AND ADMINISTERING OXYTOCIN INFUSION— continued

Intervention	Rationale
12. Notify the physician to evaluate client when oxytocin infusion is 10 mU/min. Note: A client seldom requires more than 20 to 40 mU/min of oxytocin to achieve progressive cervical dilation; 90% of clients will respond to 16 mU or less.	12. Assesses client's response to oxytocin.
13. Accurately record fluid intake and output every 2 hours.	13. Ensures proper hydration and to rule out fluid retention due to antidiuretic action of oxytocin.

CESAREAN DELIVERY

CURRENT REASONS FOR CESAREAN DELIVERY

Breech presentation
Macrosmia (fetus greater than 4000 g)
Herpes genitalis
Placental insufficiency
Severe preeclampsia or eclampsia with unripe cervix
Multiple gestation
Failure to progress in labor
Fetal distress as indicated by fetal heart rate pattern, acid base balance
Hydrocephaly

MATERNAL RISKS IN CESAREAN BIRTH

Maternal mortality, although rare, is four times higher with cesarean delivery than with vaginal delivery. Half of this increased mortality is due to complications leading to the cesarean or to maternal disease. The other half is due to the surgery itself.

Maternal mortality in repeat cesarean is about twice that in vaginal deliveries.

Maternal morbidity is much greater after cesarean; the major risks
are from:
  Infection of uterus and other genital tract structures
  Infection of respiratory or urinary tract
  Hemorrhage
Postoperative discomforts occur frequently, including incisional
  pain, gas, weakness, and difficulty in movement.
Maternal–infant bonding is interfered with through common hos-
  pital practices such as:
  General anesthesia during surgery
  Separation of mother and infant during recovery and first day
  Analgesics given the mother for pain relief
  Isolation necessary for infections
Development of mothering skills is interfered with because of
  Disorientation following anesthesia and surgery
  Pain limiting activities and requiring sedation
  Weakness, which limits the energy the mother can give to infant
    caretaking
  Postoperative complications further reducing mother–infant
    contact
  Emotional turmoil and the need to process feelings (anger, loss,
    confusion, fear, inadequacy, etc.) associated with undergoing
    cesarean birth and operative procedures
  Delay and increased difficulty gaining a sense of mastery over
    the mother's body
Breast-feeding is more difficult or impossible because of
  Pain, weakness, limited activities
  Infections or other serious complications
  Medications that may be excreted in breast milk
  Sense of inadequacy related to childbearing capabilities

GUIDELINES FOR VAGINAL DELIVERY AFTER PREVIOUS CESAREAN BIRTH*

1. Clients who have had one previous cesarean delivery with a low
   transverse incision should be counseled and encouraged to have
   a trial of labor if there are no contraindications.
2. Clients with two or more previous cesarean deliveries, with low

*From ACOG Committee Opinion No. 64, October 1988.

transverse incisions who wish to attempt vaginal birth should not be discouraged if there are no complications.

3. If no specific data on risk are available, the decision to permit a trial of labor should be assessed on an individual basis.

4. A previous classic uterine incision is a contraindication to labor.

5. Professional and institutional resources must be able to respond to acute obstetric emergencies such as performing a cesarean delivery within 30 minutes from time of decision to actual beginning of the operation.

6. Normal activity should be encouraged during latent phase of labor.

7. A physician who is capable of evaluating labor and performing a cesarean delivery must be readily available.

8. Use of oxytocin (Pitocin) for augmentation of labor for clients who have had a previous cesarean section with a low transverse incision causes no greater risk than for the general population.

9. There is no evidence that epidural anesthesia is contraindicated in these clients.

ASSESSMENT

FOCUS ASSESSMENT

Observe couple's response to being informed of the need for cesarean delivery.

Note nonverbal signs of emotional stress and level of coping.

Determine level of understanding of the reasons for the physician's decision to operate, e.g., fetal hazard, expectations for the surgery itself, and the outcomes.

Identify current level of knowledge regarding expected preoperative procedures, e.g., insertion of indwelling catheter, intravenous infusion, anesthesia.

Explore individual concerns.

Explore nonverbal indicators of feelings towards self, e.g., affect, mood, appearance, body language.

Elicit information regarding client's perception of the event, i.e., surgery, and its outcome, her self-care and infant care abilities, and future childbearing options.

Note interactions with infant, family, and visitors.

INTERVENTION

PREOPERATIVE PREPARATION

Intervention

1. When client reports to the hospital the day before surgery for preadmission testing, obtain complete blood count, type, and screen and perform initial data base assessment. Anesthesiologist performs anesthesia assessment.

2. Instruct client to take nothing by mouth after 12 midnight.

3. Remind client to report to hospital 2 hours prior to scheduled surgery time for cesarean section.

4. Assist into bed; assess vital signs.

5. Shave abdomen.

6. Insert indwelling catheter and attach to drainage bag.

7. Start intravenous fluid.

8. Remove client's jewelry for safe keeping.

9. Have client remove fingernail polish, dentures, glasses, and contact lenses.

10. Apply fetal monitor for a brief time.

Rationale

1. Completion prior to admission permits the mother to be at home with her family the night before surgery, which may increase her comfort.

2. Decreases potential for aspiration pneumonia during surgery.

3. Permits time to prepare.

4. Ensures vital signs are normal.

5. Minimizes risk of infection.

6. Keep bladder empty due to close proximity of incision.

7. Hydrates and increases maternal circulatory volume.

8. Avoids being lost.

9. Nail polish is removed so nail beds can be assessed for color. Prostheses are removed to avoid client injury.

10. Ensures that baseline FHR is normal and no decelerations are noted indicating fetal well-being.

PREOPERATIVE PREPARATION—continued

Intervention	**Rationale**
11. Administer regional anesthesia (spinal or epidural).	11. Ensures no pain is experienced.
12. Check blood pressure.	12. Ensures no hypotension is present.
13. Assist client on to operating table so there is displacement of uterus from left to right.	13. Minimizes risk of maternal hypotension resulting in decreased uteroplacental perfusion and fetal hypoxia.
14. Seat husband or significant other at head of client.	14. Provides support and sharing of childbearing experience.

OPTIONS TO FACILITATE FAMILY-CENTERED CESAREAN BIRTHS*

1. Admission to the hospital on the morning of the birth for elective cesareans so that parents can spend the previous night together (provided they have had previous orientation)
2. Father to remain with the mother during the physical preparation, e.g., shave, catheterization
3. The choice of regional anesthesia where possible, and explanation of the difference between regional and general anesthesia
4. Father in the delivery room when either regional or general anesthesia is the choice
5. Mirror or ongoing commentary from a staff member for mother or father
6. Photographs or video taken in the delivery room—if even one parent is unable to witness the birth
7. Mother's hand freed from restraint for contact with husband and infant

---

Adapted from Leach L, Sproule V: Meeting the challenge of cesarean births. JOGN 13(3):193, 1984.
*In an effort to make the cesarean delivery more family centered, the above options should be available where safety permits.

8. Opportunity for both parents to interact with the infant in the delivery room or postanesthetic recovery room
9. Opportunity for breast-feeding in the delivery room or post-anesthetic recovery room
10. Modified Leboyer practices, for example, father to submerge infant in warm water until relaxed and alert in the delivery room or in the nursery, if available for vaginal delivery
11. Delayed antimicrobials in infant's eyes
12. If father chooses not to be in the delivery room:
    (a) A support person should replace him at the mother's side
    (b) Father to be given infant to hold en route to nursery
    (c) Father to have the birth experience relayed to him by a staff member
13. Father to accompany infant to the nursery and remain with infant until both are reunited with the mother
14. Family reunited in postanesthetic recovery room if possible
15. Father to be in postanesthetic recovery room to tell his wife about the birth if she has had a general anesthetic
16. If it is difficult to reunite the family in postanesthetic delivery room, the mother's condition should be judged individually to allow the family to be reunited as soon as possible
17. Infant's condition to be judged individually so that time alone in an incubator in the nursery can be avoided if possible
18. Provision of time alone for the family in those first critical hours
19. Mother-infant nursing as soon as possible, that is, if mother feels well enough she may be able to have mother-infant nursing on the first day
20. Father to be included in the teaching of caretaking skills
21. Siblings to be included where possible

NURSING CARE PLAN

CESAREAN DELIVERY

ANXIETY, FEAR—RELATED TO CONCERN ABOUT MATERNAL AND FETAL OUTCOME, PAIN, LACK OF KNOWLEDGE ABOUT PREOPERATIVE PROCEDURES

Goals (expected outcomes)	Interventions	Rationale	Evaluation
Client/couple will verbalize her/their fears and concerns, use effective coping mechanisms to manage anxiety, and demonstrate increasing psychologic comfort.	Encourage father to remain with client as long as possible.	Provides emotional support for mother.	Father is present; couple demonstrates effective coping patterns throughout preparation and wait for surgery.
	Encourage or reinforce use of relaxation and breathing techniques to cope with preparation for surgery.	Facilitates pain management and supports effective coping with stress.	Client is relaxed and cooperative during preoperative preparations.
	Reassure regarding fetal status as possible.	Reduces anxiety for safety of fetus.	Verbalizes minimum anxiety and concern.
	Describe and explain the what, when, why, and how for all procedures as needed.	Ensures understanding of what is happening and the benefits of the procedures to reduce anxiety.	Verbalizes understanding of procedures.

Continued

NURSING CARE PLAN

CESAREAN DELIVERY—continued

Goals (expected outcomes)	Interventions	Rationale	Evaluation
ANXIETY, FEAR—RELATED TO CONCERN ABOUT MATERNAL AND FETAL OUTCOME, PAIN, LACK OF KNOWLEDGE ABOUT PREOPERATIVE PROCEDURES—cont'd			
	Describe personnel who will be present during the surgery and their roles.	Reduces anxiety at sight of unknown persons; increases confidence in care and safety.	Displays minimum anxiety.
	Encourage prepared father's presence during surgery.	Provides emotional support for mother. Reassures father of her safety and that of the infant. Permits sharing of the childbearing experience.	Father is present during surgery. Couple exhibits effective coping patterns throughout the procedure.
	Request escort for father.	Provides emotional support for him; minimizes risk of potential injury.	
KNOWLEDGE DEFICIT—REGARDING REASONS FOR SURGICAL DELIVERY, PREOPERATIVE PROCEDURES, PAIN RELIEF			
Client/couple will verbalize understanding of reasons for surgery and expected	Review information discussed in childbirth education classes.	Revives and reinforces previous discussions.	Client/couple asks questions as necessary for clarification.

effects and benefits of preoperative procedures and anesthesia.		
Explain all procedures and sensations client may experience.	Increases understanding and reduces anxiety.	Client/couple verbalizes understanding regarding reasons for surgical delivery, preoperative procedures, and method of pain management.
Emphasize benefits to mother and fetus.	Promotes perceptions of positive aspects of care procedures.	
Introduce other personnel, e.g., nurses, technicians, anesthesiologist and their roles.	Enables understanding of actions observed before and during surgery. Increases confidence in care and reduces anxiety.	Couple is calm and cooperative throughout preparation for surgery. Couple appears comfortable with decision.
Inform couple that infant will remain with them for bonding as long as status permits.	Reassures against any unnecessary interference with bonding behaviors.	

Continued

Nursing Care Plan

Cesarean Delivery—continued

SELF-ESTEEM DISTURBANCE—RELATED TO SELF-PERCEIVED "FAILURE" TO HAVE ANTICIPATED VAGINAL BIRTH, LACK OF PERSONAL "CONTROL" OVER CHILDBEARING AND TIME REQUIRED FOR RECOVERY, ALTERED BODY IMAGE

Goals (expected outcomes)	Interventions	Rationale	Evaluation
Client will identify positive aspects of self. Client will verbalize comfort with decision for surgery and satisfaction with outcome.	Avoid using terms that suggest any "failure."	Client may perceive terms such as "failure to progress" as inferring her personal control over the ability to deliver vaginally.	When expressing disappointment at change in birthing plans, client also verbalizes understanding that reasons for surgical delivery were beyond her personal control.
	Demonstrate acceptance, reassurance, and a non-judgmental attitude about comments and behaviors that indicate disappointment over having to change childbirth plans. Include father in discussions.	Communicates understanding and acceptance of her/their feelings as normal and expected. Reassures that they have not failed.	Client verbalizes the potential for vaginal birth with subsequent pregnancies.

Reassure client/couple that they managed the labor appropriately and effectively.	Provides an objective measure of their behaviors.	Couple expresses positive feelings about the care and management of the labor and delivery and satisfaction with the outcome.
Comment on their effective coping with unexpected stress.	Supports positive self-concept.	
Discuss potential for later transient depression over unfulfilled birth plans.	Anticipatory guidance enables recognition and understanding of "baby blues" as a normal phenomenon that may precipitate grieving over the inability to achieve their goal. Facilitates coping with feelings.	Client experiences minimal depression over change in birth plans and copes effectively if it occurs and recovers rapidly. Father recognizes and understands her behavior and provides needed support.

Chapter 8

THIRD AND FOURTH STAGES OF LABOR

The third stage of labor begins when the infant is delivered and completed with the delivery of the placenta.

The four stage begins after the placenta is delivered and ends when the mother's physical status has been stabilized. This stage is a transitional period for the new parents and many important physical and psychosocial tasks begin at this time.

THIRD STAGE OF LABOR

SIGNS OF PLACENTAL SEPARATION

1. The uterus becomes globular and firmer.
2. The uterus rises upward in the abdomen.
3. The umbilical cord descends 3 inches or more farther out of the vagina.
4. A sudden gush of blood often occurs.

These signs usually occur within 5 minutes after the delivery of the infant.

SUMMARY OF DELIVERY INFORMATION TO BE DOCUMENTED

The following information is noted and documented on the delivery record:

1. Date and time of delivery.
2. Presence of nuchal cord (cord around the neck or shoulder).
3. Position at delivery (OA is most common).
4. Episiotomy (type or extension, lacerations).
5. Sex of newborn.
6. Apgar scores at 1 and 5 minutes of age.
7. Response of newborn during initial care.
8. Time of placenta delivery (method, spontaneous, expressed).
9. Appearance and intactness of placenta.
10. Number of vessels in cord.
11. Any medications given to mother, i.e., oxytocin (Pitocin).
12. General condition of mother and newborn.
13. Medication given to the infant, i.e., erythromycin (Ilotycin) eye ointment.

FOURTH STAGE OF LABOR

EPISIOTOMY

Advantages

1. Ensures a straight, clean-cut surgical incision and allows easier repair and better healing.
2. Direction of opening can be controlled.
3. Avoids undue stretching and tearing of perineal musculature.
4. Shortens duration of second stage of labor.
5. Can minimize potential for later relaxed pelvic floor.
6. Heals more rapidly than a laceration.
7. Facilitates delivery of a distressed infant.

Disadvantages

1. Pain.
2. Increased risk of infection.
3. Inability to void and defecate after delivery because of pain and edema.
4. Increased risk for dyspareunia (may last 6 months or more).

CLASSIFICATION OF PERINEAL LACERATIONS

First Degree Laceration: Involves the fourchette, perineal skin, and vaginal mucous membrane without involving the muscles.

Second Degree Laceration: Involves (in addition to skin and mucous membrane) the muscles of the perineal body but not the rectal spincter. These tears usually extend upward on one or both sides of the vagina.

Third Degree Laceration: Extends completely through the skin, mucous membrane, and rectal spincter.

Fourth Degree Laceration: Extends through the rectal mucosa into the rectum.

ASSESSMENT

INITIAL MATERNAL POSTPARTUM ASSESSMENT

1. Vital signs
   Blood pressure
   Pulse
   Respiration
2. Fundus
   Height
   Size
   Location
   Consistency
   Massage initiated if relaxation occurs
3. Lochia
   Amount
   Consistency
   Color
   Odor
4. Perineal status
   Episiotomy
   Tears
   Edema
   Discoloration
   Bleeding
   Hematoma present
5. Bladder status
   Distention
   Foley in place if cesarean delivery
6. Intravenous fluid
   Site
   Type
   Bottle number
   Amount infused
   Medication(s) added to IV (e.g., Pitocin)
   Amount remaining in bottle or bag
7. Anesthesia
   Type
   Motor or sensory residual remaining
8. Parents' reactions and responses to the newborn
   Do they look at or away
   What do they say
   Do they reach for or push away
9. Pain
   Source (episiotomy, afterpains, cesarean delivery incision)

Sample Narrative Charting: T 98.2 (F) BP 100/70, pulse 80 and respirations 18. Fundus at the U, firm, midline. Massaged, no blood or clots expressed. Bleeding moderate, presently bright red. Perineum intact, no edema or bruising noted. Ice pack in place. No bladder distention palpable. #3 IV (1000 ml Normasol with 10U Pitocin added) infusing at 125 ml/hr. States, "My bottom is beginning to burn a little but I still want to breast-feed my baby." Both parents are inspecting infant carefully, exclaiming how beautiful and alert it is. Infant smacking lips and sucking on fingers and fists. Is holding one of father's fingers.

FOCUS ASSESSMENT

Monitor pulse, respirations, and blood pressure closely.

Monitor consistency and height of fundus, amount and character of lochia every 15 minutes for 1 hour, then every 30 minutes for 1 hour.

Note verbal and nonverbal signs of pain.

Identify signs and symptoms of fatigue.

Monitor intake and output.

Elicit verbalization of perception of birth experience.

Observe interaction with newborn and significant other.

Identify individual teaching or learning needs.

ONGOING ASSESSMENT DURING FOURTH STAGE

Ongoing assessments are done every 15 minutes during the first hour and every 30 minutes during the second hour after delivery. Temperature is taken once within the first postpartum hour. Vaginal bleeding is assessed for amount, color, consistency, and presence of clots or foul odor. During each assessment the fundus is massaged to ensure that bleeding is not excessive and its location, height, and consistency are documented.

1. Vital signs
   Temperature
   Blood pressure
   Pulse
   Respirations
2. Fundus
   Height
   Location
   Consistency
3. Lochia
   Amount
   Consistency
   Odor
4. Perineal status
   Episiotomy
   Tears
   Edema
   Discoloration
   Bleeding
   Hematoma
5. Bladder status
   Distention
   Foley patent (if used)
   Output
   Urine color
6. Pain
   Source
7. Intravenous fluids
   Type
   Bottle or bag number
   Amount infused
   Medication(s) added
   Amount remaining in bottle or bag
   IV site
8. Residual effects of anesthesia
   Motor or sensory
9. Parental responses to newborn
   Success with breast-feeding
      (if chosen feeding method)
   Face-to-face interaction

STANDARDIZED RECORDING OF VAGINAL FLOW

1. Scant—blood noted on tissue after wiping or less than 1-inch stain on peripad
2. Light—less than 4-inch stain on peripad
3. Moderate—less than 6-inch stain on peripad
4. Heavy—peripad saturated within 1 hour; bleeding is bright red and clots may be present

DEVIATIONS FROM EXPECTED PATTERNS DURING IMMEDIATE POSTPARTUM PERIOD

The following assessment findings should be reported to the physician immediately:

1. Uterine atony
2. Excessive bleeding
3. Hypotension or tachycardia
4. Hypertension
5. Headache or visual disturbance
6. Elevated temperature

TRANSFERRING MOTHER TO POSTPARTUM CARE

The postpartum unit is notified that the client is ready to be transferred. The mother is transported to the postpartum unit by bed or wheelchair.

The following information is to be communicated by the transferring recovery (labor and delivery) nurse to the receiving postpartum unit nurse when the mother is transferred from the recovery area to the postpartum unit.

Report Information

1. Review prenatal history relevant to postpartum care:
   Any known allergies
   Mother's Rh status
   Any problems during pregnancy
   If mother was term
2. Review events of labor and delivery:
   Normal or abnormal length of labor
   Mother's response to labor
   FHR response during labor
   Analgesia or anesthesia
   Vaginal or cesarean delivery
   Spontaneous or forceps delivery
3. Review recovery events:
   Fundal location and status
   Lochia description
   Vital signs
   Bladder status
   Perineal trauma (if any)
   Bonding events

NURSING CARE PLAN

FOURTH STAGE OF LABOR

Goals (expected outcomes)	Interventions	Rationale	Evaluation
PAIN—RELATED TO EPISIOTOMY			
Client will experience minimum pain.	Apply ice (in bag or glove) to perineum.	Ice numbs area.	Client verbalizes she is more comfortable.
	Administer analgesia for episiotomy pain and afterpains as needed.	Medication should minimize pain so that family interaction can occur.	
SLEEP PATTERN DISTURBANCE—RELATED TO EXHAUSTIVE WORK OF LABOR			
Client will be rested and sleep after bonding time with infant.	Assist to position of comfort.	Promotes rest and facilitates interaction with infant.	Family displays positive interactions with infant.
	Provide quiet, relaxing environment conducive to rest and bonding; ensure privacy.	Promotes rest and facilitates interaction with infant.	Client is quiet and relaxed as she interacts with her "new" family.
			Client sleeps after bonding time.
ALTERED NUTRITION—RELATED TO FASTING OF LABOR			
Client will tolerate fluids and have a healthy appetite.	Encourage fluids (cold or warm if desired).	Labor requires great energy expenditure. Mother usually very	Client is tolerating fluids well. Intake 500 ml warm sweetened tea.

			thirsty. Fluids should be given initially to ensure no gastric upset.	Client eats 80% of regular diet and verbalizes relief of hunger and thirst.

FLUID VOLUME DEFICIT—RELATED TO EXCESSIVE BLOOD LOSS SECONDARY TO UTERINE ATONY, CERVICAL AND/OR VAGINAL LACERATIONS

Client will exhibit moderate amount of lochia rubra.	Massage fundus as needed to maintain firmness and expel clots.	Stimulates uterine contractions, which compress vessels in placenta site. Minimizes blood loss. Clots may interfere with firmness and contribute to increase in size of uterus leading to relaxation.	Uterus well contracted, midline in position, at level of umbilicus. No clots present. Moderate amount of lochia rubra.
	Encourage to void.	Full bladder contributes to uterine relaxation.	Bladder not distended.
	Change pads after every fundal check.	Allows estimation of blood loss.	Blood (lochia) loss is minimal to moderate. Vital signs are normal (compared to prenatal and labor and delivery).

Continued

Nursing Care Plan

Fourth Stage of Labor—continued

Self-Disturbance—Related to Unfulfilled Birth Plans

Goals (expected outcomes)	Interventions	Rationale	Evaluation
Client will integrate a positive birthing experience.	Encourage verbalization of labor and delivery experience. Reinforce positive view of performance.	Time of openness and nurse can reinforce positive interactions and give explanations when needed.	Family is communicating openly about their birth experience.
	Answer anticipated as well as verbalized questions about labor and delivery.	Minimizes memory gaps (missing part of experiences).	Client discusses the labor and delivery experience and asks questions about areas that are unclear or cannot be remembered.
	Facilitate family interactions.		Family talking about the experience. Include nurse as integral part of experience.
	Praise the couple on how well they managed.	Accentuate the positive—"Did a good job." Parents need to feel supported and comfortable about the experience.	Couple emphasizes their strengths and minimizes their perceived weaknesses or disappointments.

	Encourage verbalization of negative perceptions.	Allows nurse to clarify and minimize the negative or misconception.	Open-mindedness of present may minimize negative feelings and clear up misconceptions.

ALTERED PARENTING—RELATED TO INEXPERIENCE AND FEELINGS OF INADEQUACY

Client will display readiness to begin to parent.	Encourage family interactions after delivery.	Parents need to begin to develop confidence in their new parenting role.	Couple expresses their lack of parenting skills but verbalizes their desire and readiness to parent and work on acquired skills.
	Note and communicate reciprocal responses with newborn.	Important cues of parenting role.	Bonding evidenced by eye contact, cuddling, stroking. Calls infant by name.

Chapter 9

MATERNAL NURSING CARE IN THE POSTPARTUM PERIOD

This chapter continues discussions of the postpartum period. Content focuses on nursing care of the new mother and supportive actions that assist families in successfully adapting to the new demands of parenthood. Emphasis is placed on nursing assessment of factors that influence the mother's recovery, her caregiving abilities, and her successful role transition.

ASSESSMENT

Nursing assessments of the biophysical changes that occur in the puerperium include vital signs, breast changes, condition of the abdomen, signs of uterine involution, condition of the perineum and episiotomy, urinary and intestinal elimination, and Homans' sign.

POSTPARTUM NURSING ASSESSMENT CHECKLIST

During the first 24 hours after delivery, the mother's temperature, pulse, respirations, and blood pressure are usually assessed every 4 hours.

A. Vital signs
B. Breasts
    1. Skin integrity (nipples supple; intact, reddened, fissures)
    2. Consistency (soft, firm, engorged)
    3. Lactation status (suppressed; colostrum, milk)
C. Abdomen (soft, distended, bowel sounds)
D. Involution
    1. Uterus (fundal height and consistency)
    2. Lochia (amount, character, type)
E. Perineum and perianal area (suture line, edema, pain; hemorrhoids)
F. Elimination
    1. Urinary (first three voidings, amount, color, character)
    2. Bowel (flatulence; stool)
G. Homans' sign (absent; present, right, left)
H. Other: complaint of pain or discomfort
    1. Characteristics (sharp, dull, aching)

    2. Degree of discomfort (mild, moderate, severe)
    3. Location (localized, incisional, general)
    4. Cause (precipitated by, associated with, relieved by)
I. Laboratory values
    1. Hematocrit
    2. Hemoglobin
    3. White blood count

Sample Narrative Charting

Routine Postpartum Assessment: Alert and responsive. No complaint of pain. Breasts soft. Nipples supple and intact, no evidence of redness or cracking. Fundus firm and in midline, U/1; moderate lochia rubra. Active bowel sounds present. Episiotomy clean and healing, suture line intact. Voiding Q.S. Homans' sign absent. Ambulates easily without assistance. Bonding evidenced by eye contact, stroking, snuggling; calls newborn by name.

If findings at the end of the second hour after admission to the postpartum unit are within normal limits, the intervals for subsequent assessments are lengthened gradually throughout the first 24 hours following delivery, e.g., hourly, every 2 hours.

For the remainder of the hospital stay, the nursing assessments of the postpartum mother's physical status are done once each shift.

CHARACTERISTICS OF NORMAL LOCHIA*

	Normal lochial progression				
Characteristic	**Rubra**	*to*	**Serosa**	*to*	**Alba**
Color	Dark red; may have small clots		Pinkish; thin, watery, no clots		Cream to yellowish
Odor	Similar to menstrual flow		No odor		No odor
Occurrence	Days 1 to 3		Days 4 to 10		Days 11 to 21
Amount	Moderate		Moderate to small		Scant

*The lochial pattern is characteristic of the stage of endometrial healing. Immediately following the tissue trauma of placental separation, lochia is red to dark red; as venous sinuses are constricted and healing begins, the amount of blood diminishes. Marked alterations from this pattern suggest possible inflammatory interference with normal healing processes.

POSTPARTUM HEMATOLOGIC CHANGES IN BLOOD VALUES

Blood value	Late pregnancy (37-40 weeks)	Postpartum (second day)
Hemoglobin	12.1-12.7 g/dl	10.0-11.4 g/dl
Hematocrit	35%-42%	32%-38%
Leukocytes	5000-12,000/mm	14,000-16,000/mm

The extent of changes in postpartum blood values is assessed by comparing results of samples drawn during the month preceding labor with those drawn on the second postpartum day. Samples drawn at other times cannot be used for comparison because of the following: (1) although findings of the initial blood work may be within normal limits for a healthy adult female, the mother may develop anemia during the months of gestation; (2) hematocrit values determined during labor may reflect hemoconcentration resulting from dehydration—when used as a baseline measure, they convey an erroneous impression of excessive blood loss; (3) hemodilution resulting from postpartum diuresis requires 12 to 24 hours to occur; and (4) even acute hemorrhage may not cause a significant drop in hemoglobin concentration. A drop of 1 g in the hemoglobin level or 3% in the hematocrit value reflects a blood loss of approximately 500 ml.

POSTPARTUM RISK FACTORS

Risk factor	At risk for	Assessment findings
Breast-feeding	Infection (mastitis)	Nipples red, appear irritated; nipple fissures; pain on palpation or breast-feeding
Uterine over-distention (hydramnios, large fetus, multiple pregnancy)	Uterine atony, immediate postpartum hemorrhage (within first 24 hr)	Fundus boggy; heavy lochia rubra; hypotension, tachycardia
Prolonged labor Operative (forceps) delivery	Lacerations	Bright red vaginal bleeding
	Uterine atony, hemorrhage	Fundus boggy; heavy lochia rubra

POSTPARTUM RISK FACTORS—continued

Risk factor	At risk for	Assessment findings
	Hematoma	Distended, firm, often bluish mass (labial, perineal); perineal pain
	Edema of trigone area of bladder; impaired urinary elimination	Unable to void; inadequate urinary output
Premature rupture of membranes	Infection (endometritis)	Temperature elevation, tachycardia, malaise; fundus tender to palpation; lochial change
Prolonged second stage of labor	Thrombus formation; thrombophlebitis	Presence of Homans' sign
Retained placental fragments	Delayed postpartum hemorrhage (after first 24 hr)	Bright red vaginal bleeding

INTERVENTION

CLIENT SELF-CARE EDUCATION: CHECKLIST

    I. Physical aspects of self-care
       A. Bathing and breast care, support, and comfort
          1. Breast-feeding (bra, milk expression, ice packs)
          2. Bottle-feeding (bra, ice packs)
       B. Involution: fundus and characteristic lochia; afterpains
       C. Perineal care (solutions, witch hazel pads)
          1. Sitz bath
          2. Perineal heat lamp
       D. Nutrition and hydration (breast-feeding, bottle-feeding)
       E. Rest and sleep
       F. Exercise (ambulation, postpartum and Kegel's exercises)
       G. Bowel elimination
       H. Signs to report promptly
       I. Available assistance with household tasks

CLIENT SELF-CARE EDUCATION: CHECKLIST—continued

   II. Psychosocial aspects of self-care
      A. Emotional adjustment (bonding, taking-in, taking-hold, letting-go)
         1. Self-image
         2. Baby blues
      B. Family relations
         1. Family adjustments to the new baby (parental, sibling, extended family)
         2. Role change
         3. Alterations in life-style
      C. Sexuality and family planning
      D. Visitors
   III. Infant care
      A. Feeding (breast, formula)
      B. Positioning and handling
      C. Bathing
      D. Cord and circumcision care
      E. Clothing and diapering
      F. Temperature and thermometer use
      G. Suctioning with bulb syringe
      H. Infant behavior patterns (sleeping, crying, fussing, neuromuscular control, eye movements, developmental patterns, elimination patterns)
      I. Safety (car seat use, never leaving baby alone on bed or table, nonflammable clothing)
      J. Recognizing signs of illness; signs to report promptly to physician
   IV. Community resources (La Leche International, family service agencies, local mother's support groups, parenting education sources)

CLIENT SELF-CARE EDUCATION: BREAST CARE FOR THE BREAST-FEEDING MOTHER

Action	**Rationale**
1. Wear bra 24 hr/day.	1. Maintains support; reduces discomfort from normal movement.
a. May use breast pads or clean handkerchief	a. Absorbs milk leakage; protects clothing

CLIENT SELF-CARE EDUCATION: BREAST CARE FOR THE BREAST-FEEDING MOTHER—continued

Action	Rationale
b. Avoid plastic liners or pads	b. Plastic retains body heat and moisture
c. Air dry nipples after each feeding	c. Reduces nipple irritation
2. Bathe breasts and nipples with clear water daily.	2. Soap removes natural nipple secretions, is drying, and can lead to cracking
3. Gently pat dry.	3. Friction is irritating to nipples, may traumatize tissue
4. Inspect nipples for signs of redness, cracking.	4. Facilitates early detection and prompt management of irritation; minimizes potential for infection
Sore nipples care	
a. Expose to air for 15 to 30 min several times daily	a. Reduces nipple irritation; promotes healing
b. Express colostrum and rub over nipple area	b. Colostrum is very healing
c. If ordered, may use hydrous lanolin	c. Soothing
d. Alternate breast for start of each feeding	d. Vigorous sucking is most pronounced at beginning of feeding
e. Check that most of areola is in infant's mouth	e. Distributes sucking pressures; protects nipple
f. Change nursing positions with each feeding	f. Subjects different nipple areas to stress of sucking
5. Examine breasts after each feeding.	5. Reveals signs of infection
Signs to report promptly NOTIFY PRIMARY HEALTH CARE PROVIDER IF THE FOLLOWING OCCUR:	
a. Acute tenderness or pain	Usually involves only one breast; may occur in either breast or both breasts may be involved
b. Local or general redness, heat, swelling	
c. General feeling of malaise	
d. Marked rise in body temperature	
e. Chills	*Continued*

CLIENT SELF-CARE EDUCATION: BREAST CARE FOR THE BREAST-FEEDING MOTHER—continued

Action	Rationale
6. Engorgement.	
a. Massage breasts with gentle, downward milking motion; may be done during shower	a. Increases circulation, opens lacteal ducts; expresses milk
b. May apply ice packs for 15 to 20 min between nursing periods	b. Reduces discomfort by decreasing circulation to breast(s)
7. *Discontinuing breast-feeding*	
a. Do not massage breasts or express milk to relieve discomfort	a. Stimulates further milk production; prolongs lactation
b. May apply ice packs for 15 to 20 min several times daily	b. Relieves discomfort
c. Wear well-fitting bra 24 hours each day until discomfort subsides	c. Minimizes pain from movement; provides support to breasts that have become larger and heavier during pregnancy and engorgement
d. May take aspirin or acetaminophen for pain as directed by primary health care provider	d. Analgesia; discomfort usually lasts 1 to 2 days
e. May drink to satisfy thirst but avoid excessive amounts of fluids	e. Excessive fluid may increase engorgement

EVALUATION

DISCHARGE ASSESSMENT TOOL: EARLY DISCHARGE: SAMPLE CHECKLIST

1. The client had a normal, uncomplicated term pregnancy (38 to 42 weeks gestation).
2. On admission hemoglobin and hematocrit levels were within normal limits.
3. The client had normal, uncomplicated labor and vaginal delivery; no excessive blood loss.

DISCHARGE ASSESSMENT TOOL: EARLY DISCHARGE: SAMPLE CHECKLIST—continued

4. All assessment findings were within normal limits.
   a. Mother
      (1) Vital signs stable
      (2) Firm fundus
      (3) Moderate lochia rubra
      (4) Perineum intact, no evidence of hematoma
      (5) Homans' sign absent
      (6) Voiding spontaneously in adequate amounts
      (7) Tolerating fluids without nausea or vomiting
      (8) Ambulating without assistance; not weak or dizzy
   b. Infant
      (1) Appropriate for gestational age (>2500 g)
      (2) Vital signs stable; no excessive mucus
      (3) Normal cry and reflexes
      (4) Sucking well during initial feeding(s)
      (5) Initial voiding and stool observed
      (6) Coombs' test negative (if mother Rh negative and infant Rh positive)
      (7) Normal cord blood bilirubin level (if ordered)
   c. Signs of positive parental attachment
5. Appointment made for office visit within 48-72 hr (or scheduled home visit by nurse within 48-72 hr of discharge).
6. Client teaching has been completed.
   a. Accurate return-demonstrations of the following:
      (1) Self fundal check
      (2) Perineal care
      (3) Basic infant care (diapering, cord care)
   b. Verbal and written postpartum instructions provided
      (1) Self-care, infant care procedures
      (2) Limitations on activities
      (3) Signs to be reported promptly to primary health care provider
   c. Provided with important telephone numbers
      (1) Obstetrician or nurse midwife, pediatrician
      (2) Hospital maternity unit
      (3) Emergency medical service agency

NURSING CARE PLAN

IMMEDIATE POSTPARTUM PERIOD (FIRST 24 HOURS)

Goals (expected outcomes)	Interventions	Rationale	Evaluation
POTENTIAL FLUID VOLUME DEFICIT (2)—RELATED TO EXCESSIVE BLEEDING			
Client will adapt successfully to anatomic and physiologic changes of immediate postpartum period without incident.	Perform gentle fundal massage if necessary to firm boggy uterus.	Stimulates uterine muscle to contract; minimizes blood loss (see also Nursing Procedure: Fundus Check; Emergency Nursing Intervention: Immediate Postpartum Hemorrhage: Fundal Massage).	Condition is stable on all status Vital signs Fundus firm, U/U, in abdominal midline Moderate lochia rubra
	Express clots from uterus.	Empties uterus, allows effective contractions; enables estimate of blood loss.	
	Report and record any deviations from normal patterns.	Enables prompt medical or nursing intervention.	
	Encourage voiding.	Distended bladder interferes with effective uterine contractions that close endometrial vessels at placental site.	Voids spontaneously

ALTERED PATTERNS OF URINARY ELIMINATION—RELATED TO POSTPARTUM DIURESIS

Client will void spontaneously to empty bladder within 6-8 hr after delivery.	Encourage client to drink warm fluids as tolerated.	Re-establishes hydration; encourages relaxation.	Voids 300 ml spontaneously on first three occasions.
	Promote relaxation.	Promotes comfort and relaxation.	
	Administer analgesics if indicated.	"Normal" surroundings and anatomic position encourage voiding.	
	Position client for comfort.		
	Assist to bathroom or bedside commode.		

URINARY RETENTION (ACUTE)—RELATED TO BLADDER EDEMA SECONDARY TO TRAUMA DURING DELIVERY

	Provide perineal care with warm solution.	Stimulates voiding, promotes comfort and healing; minimizes potential for autoinfection.	Fundus firm, in abdominal midline, U/U; moderate lochia rubra.
	Measure first three voidings.	Provides estimate of adequacy of emptying bladder.	
	Perform fundal check.	Reduces potential for excessive bleeding.	

Continued

NURSING CARE PLAN

IMMEDIATE POSTPARTUM PERIOD (FIRST 24 HOURS)—continued

Goals (expected outcomes)	Interventions	Rationale	Evaluation
URINARY RETENTION (ACUTE)—RELATED TO BLADDER EDEMA SECONDARY TO TRAUMA DURING DELIVERY—cont'd			
	Catheterize for bladder distention, inability to void or empty.	Empties bladder, prevents distention; allows return of normal bladder tone.	
ALTERED FAMILY PROCESSES—RELATED TO ROLE CHANGE, TAKING-IN, AND TAKING-HOLD			
Client will demonstrate attachment behaviors, e.g., bonding with newborn.	Place stable infant in mother's arms. Provide privacy for new family.	Encourages attachment and bonding.	Demonstrates bonding behaviors Eye contact Stroking Cuddling Calls by name
Client will begin integration of newborn into family unit.	Encourage both parents to interact with infant. Reduce light in room. Assist with initial breast-feeding if necessary.	Encourages infant to open eyes and interact with parents. Encourages bonding, later success in breast-feeding; stimulates uterine contractions.	Appears happy and comfortable with newborn

NORMAL POST PARTUM

Goals (expected outcomes)	Interventions	Rationale	Evaluation
	Encourage active participation in and assumption of responsibility for infant care; meet needs or guidance and assistance.	Introduces basic infant care concepts and skills in supportive environment; facilitates development of parental confidence and competence in infant care skills.	Demonstrates growing confidence in own abilities to provide care.
PAIN—RELATED TO BREAST ENGORGEMENT SECONDARY TO IMPENDING LACTATION			
Client will demonstrate understanding and applications of client teaching.	Perform client teaching. Explain causes. Discuss comfort measures.	Establishes shared knowledge base; encourages active participation in pain management (See also Client Self-Care Education: Breast Care for the Breast-Feeding Mother).	On request, accurately explains comfort measures and rationale in own words.
Client will experience relief of discomfort.			Return-demonstrates procedures.
			Complies with nursing recommendations.
			Verbalizes relief of discomfort.
			Displays no nonverbal evidence of pain.

Continued

NURSING CARE PLAN

NORMAL POST PARTUM—continued

Goals (expected outcomes)	Interventions	Rationale	Evaluation
PAIN—RELATED TO BREAST ENGORGEMENT SECONDARY TO IMPENDING LACTATION—cont'd			
	Recommend mother wear bra at all times.	Provides support, minimizes movement and discomfort of engorged breasts.	
	Explain benefit of warm packs or shower before feeding.	Heat increases circulation, facilitates expression of milk.	
	Demonstrate how to express milk.	Reduces pressure and discomfort from engorgement.	
	Discuss feeding techniques (frequency, length, infant position).	Encourages successful breast-feeding; minimizes potential for problems related to nursing.	
AFTERPAINS SECONDARY TO UTERINE CONTRACTIONS ASSOCIATED WITH BREAST-FEEDING			
	Explain prevention (analgesic 15 to 30 min before feeding; empty bladder).	Promotes comfort (See also Client Self-Care Education: Afterpains).	

| | Discuss fundal massage, prone position, leg lifts after feeding. | Promotes comfort and healing (see also Client Self-Care Education: Perineal Care; Nursing Procedure: Perineal Lamp). | |

PERINEAL TENDERNESS SECONDARY TO EPISIOTOMY

| | Discuss and demonstrate perineal care, use of sitz bath/perineal lamp. Describe tensing gluteal muscles on sitting. | Enables mother to participate actively in own care, minimize potential for infection. | |

POTENTIAL FOR INFECTION—RELATED TO IMPAIRED SKIN INTEGRITY, BREAST (MASTITIS), SECONDARY TO NIPPLE FISSURES ASSOCIATED WITH BREAST-FEEDING

| Client will demonstrate understanding and application of client teaching. Client will minimize potential for infection. Client will experience uneventful recovery. | Perform client teaching. Explain causes. Discuss prevention. Describe early signs of infection. | Enables mother to participate actively in own care, minimize potential for infection; facilitates early identification and treatment of infection. | On request, accurately explains preventive measures in own words. Return-demonstrates procedures. Complies with nursing recommendations. |

Continued

NURSING CARE PLAN

NORMAL POST PARTUM—continued

Goals (expected outcomes)	Interventions	Rationale	Evaluation
POTENTIAL FOR INFECTION—RELATED TO IMPAIRED SKIN INTEGRITY, BREAST (MASTITIS), SECONDARY TO NIPPLE FISSURES ASSOCIATED WITH BREAST-FEEDING—cont'd			
	Advise client to: Avoid soap; bathe breasts with clear water only. Air dry nipples after nursing. Avoid use of plastic bra liners, nipple shields. Apply lanolin after feeding as directed.	Minimizes potential for dry skin, nipple fissures (see also Client Self-Care Education: Breast Care for the Breast-Feeding Mother).	Exhibits no signs or symptoms of infection (e.g., afebrile).
TRAUMA TO UTERINE ENDOMETRIUM (ENDOMETRITIS) SECONDARY TO PLACENTAL SEPARATION			
	Discuss and demonstrate perineal care, pad change, handwashing.	Minimizes potential for autoinfection (see also Client Self-Care Education: Perineal Care).	
IMPAIRED SKIN INTEGRITY, PERINEAL (WOUND INFECTION), SECONDARY TO EPISIOTOMY			
	Discuss perineal care, pad change, handwashing.	Promotes comfort and healing; minimizes potential for autoinfection.	

CONSTIPATION—RELATED TO REDUCED INTESTINAL MOTILITY

Client will re-establish normal bowel elimination pattern.	Perform client teaching: Encourage early ambulation. Encourage free intake of fluids (water 6-8 glasses daily). Encourage intake of fresh fruits, bran, vegetables. Reassure client about lack of discomfort accompanying stool expulsion. Administer stool softener as ordered.	Encourages peristalsis; reduces potential for constipation; minimizes risk of discomfort related to hard, packed stool.	Complies with nursing recommendations. Has spontaneous expulsion of normal stool.

SLEEP PATTERN DISTURBANCE—RELATED TO INTERRUPTED REST SECONDARY TO BREAST-FEEDING

Client will maximize time for rest and sleep.	Perform client teaching: Limit visitors and calls to specific times during day.	Engenders rest and reduces energy expenditures resulting from "hostessing" (see also	Complies with nursing recommendations. Rests and sleeps during day.

Continued

NURSING CARE PLAN

NORMAL POST PARTUM—continued

Goals (expected outcomes)	Interventions	Rationale	Evaluation
SLEEP PATTERN DISTURBANCE—RELATED TO INTERRUPTED REST SECONDARY TO BREAST-FEEDING—cont'd			
			Verbalizes feeling refreshed.
	Nap while baby sleeps. Rest frequently during day. Retire early. Organize nursing care to facilitate adequate rest.	Client Self-Care Education: Rest and Sleep). Encourages rest and relaxation; reduces potential for sleep deficit.	
ALTERED FAMILY PROCESSES—RELATED TO ROLE CHANGE, TAKING-IN, AND TAKING-HOLD			
Client will demonstrate attachment behaviors, e.g., bonding with newborn.	Place stable infant in mother's arms. Provide privacy for new family.	Encourages attachment and bonding.	Demonstrates bonding behaviors: Eye contact Stroking Cuddling Calling infant by name
Client will begin integration of newborn into family unit.	Encourage both parents to interact with infant. Reduce light in room.	Encourages infant to open eyes and interact with parents.	Appears happy and comfortable with newborn.

	Assist with initial breast-feeding if necessary.	Encourages bonding, later success in breast-feeding; stimulates uterine contractions.	Demonstrates growing confidence in own abilities to provide care.
	Encourage active participation in and assumption of responsibility for infant care. Meet needs for guidance and assistance.	Introduces basic infant care concepts and skills in supportive environment; facilitates development of parental confidence and competence in infant care skills.	

KNOWLEDGE DEFICIT (LEARNING NEED)—REGARDING HEALTH MAINTENANCE, SELF-ASSESSMENT OF BREASTS, NIPPLES, INVOLUTION, EPISIOTOMY, SIGNS OF POSTPARTUM COMPLICATIONS

Client will demonstrate understanding and application of client teaching. Client will actively participate in her own health maintenance. Client will identify early signs of postpartum complications.	Perform client teaching: Explain reasons for self-assessment. Discuss and demonstrate each component of postpartum assessment. Breasts and nipples Fundal check (height and consistency)	Enables active client participation in own health maintenance.	On request, explains assessment and rationale. Accurately return-demonstrates assessment of: Breasts and nipples Involution progress Lochial volume and character Healing progress of surgical wound

Continued

Nursing Care Plan

Normal Post Partum—continued

Goals (expected outcomes)	Interventions	Rationale	Evaluation
KNOWLEDGE DEFICIT (LEARNING NEED)—REGARDING HEALTH MAINTENANCE, SELF-ASSESSMENT OF BREASTS, NIPPLES, INVOLUTION, EPISIOTOMY, SIGNS OF POSTPARTUM COMPLICATIONS—cont'd			
	Lochia (amount and color)		Describes signs and symptoms to report promptly to primary health care provider.
	Signs of healing surgical wound		Experiences an uneventful recovery.
	Describe and discuss signs to report to primary health care provider.	Encourages early diagnosis of emerging health problems (see also Client Self-Care Education: Breast Care for the Breast-Feeding Mother; Client Self-Care Education: Involution).	
SELF-CARE ACTIVITIES			
Client will gain knowledge and skills needed for implementing effective postpartum self-care.	Perform client teaching: Breast care Perineal care Heat therapy	Enables active client participation in own health maintenance; minimizes potential for postpartum complications.	Verbalizes understanding of principles and self-care procedures. Performs self-care actions

Client will develop competence and comfort in performing self-care procedures. Client will develop confidence in own abilities. Client will assume responsibility for self-care.	Nutrition, hydration Elimination Exercise, rest, sleep Prevention of infection Encourages and supports positive self-concept.	appropriately; displays no evidence of anxiety. Verbalizes and demonstrates confidence in own ability.
INFANT CARE Client will gain knowledge and skills necessary for safe, effective infant care. Client will develop competence in performing basic infant care procedures. Client will develop confidence in own abilities to provide safe, effective infant care. Client will assume responsibility for basic infant care.	Perform client teaching: Feeding Burping Suctioning with bulb syringe Bathing Cord care Circumcision care Diapering Enables client to perform basic infant care procedures effectively. Reduces anxiety; engenders confidence in own abilities. Encourages and supports positive self-concept.	Verbalizes understanding of principles and procedures. Performs procedures accurately. Appears relaxed and comfortable in providing basic infant care.

Continued

NURSING CARE PLAN

NORMAL POST PARTUM—continued

Goals (expected outcomes)	Interventions	Rationale	Evaluation
CONTRACEPTION			
Client will gain knowledge and understanding of selected aspects of current methods of contraception. Client will make an informed choice among available methods for family planning.	Perform client teaching: methods available Action Contraindications Advantages Disadvantages Effectiveness Risks	Enables client(s) to make an informed choice among options available for effective family planning.	Selects method appropriate to individual needs and desires. Experiences success in avoiding or achieving future pregnancy.
SEXUALITY PATTERNS—RELATED TO DYSPAREUNIA SECONDARY EPISIOTOMY			
Client will minimize potential for sexual dysfunction.	Provide anticipatory guidance: Suggest couple defer coitus until episiotomy is less sensitive to pressure (approximately 3 wk).	Enables client(s) to understand and minimize maternal discomfort (see also Client Self-Care Education: Sexuality).	Verbalizes understanding of factors that may cause discomfort.

DECREASED VAGINAL LUBRICATION SECONDARY TO LOW ESTROGEN LEVEL

Client will resume mutually satisfying sexual relationship with significant other.	Recommend use of spermicidal cream for lubrication.	Reduces friction discomfort; allows satisfaction of sexual drive.

FEAR OF PREGNANCY

Client will make an informed choice regarding method of contraception.	Suggest use of spermicidal cream during interim between discharge and postpartum check-up.	Promotes comfort; minimizes risk of unexpected pregnancy.	Identifies ways to minimize discomfort and potential for unexpected pregnancy.
	Client teaching: If desired, discuss options for family planning.	Facilitates informed decision making; encourages selection of method of contraception appropriate to individual needs and desires.	

Continued

NURSING CARE PLAN

NORMAL POST PARTUM—continued

Goals (expected outcomes)	Interventions	Rationale	Evaluation
SELF-ESTEEM DISTURBANCE—RELATED TO FEELINGS OF INADEQUACY AND INSECURITY REGARDING SELF-CARE, INFANT CARE			
Client will recognize the influence of physiologic changes on emotional status.	Provide anticipatory guidance: Discuss normal psychologic changes in the postpartum period; explain transitory nature; emphasize normalcy.	Enables client(s) to understand and accept emerging feelings; minimizes fear "something is wrong." (see also Client Self-Care Education: Psychosocial Aspects of the Postpartum Period).	Copes effectively with postpartum letdown.
ALTERED HORMONE LEVELS			
	Explain physiologic changes; emphasize transitory nature and normalcy.		
FATIGUE SECONDARY TO ALTERED LIFE-STYLE			
Client will organize activities to allow time for rest and relaxation.	Enable future coping by aiding client to develop confidence in self-care, infant care.	Enables effective coping; supports positive self-concept; minimizes symptoms.	Experiences uneventful transition to parenthood.

NEWBORN NURSING CARE

Chapter 10

IMMEDIATE CARE OF THE HEALTHY NEWBORN

The initial care of the newborn during fourth stage labor consists of four components: (1) preventing heat loss, (2) maintaining a patent airway, (3) establishing and maintaining respirations, and (4) physical evaluation.

ITEMS TO BE AVAILABLE WHEN DELIVERY IS IMMINENT

1. Preheated radiant warmer
2. Warm sterile towels, blankets, and newborn hat
3. Oxygen, suction, resuscitation equipment
4. Identification bracelets
5. Erythromycin eye ointment
6. Neonatal vitamin K (phytonadione); protect drug from light
7. Birth record, foot printer, alcohol sponges
8. Chart materials

Note: Precheck equipment to ensure everything works properly.

ASSESSMENT

THE APGAR SCORING CHART

Sign	0	1	2
Heart rate	Absent	Slow (less than 100)	Over 100
Respiratory effort	Absent	Slow, irregular	Good, crying
Muscle tone	Flaccid	Some flexion of extremities	Active motion
Reflex irritability	No response	Weak cry or grimace	Vigorous cry
Color	Blue, pale	Body pink, extremities blue	Completely pink

Each of the five signs are evaluated and given a score of 0, 1, or 2 at 1 minute and 5 minutes of age. The highest possible score is 10.

IMMEDIATE POSTDELIVERY ASSESSMENT OF THE NEWBORN*

	Assessment	Significant Findings
INSPECTION		
Head	Molding Caput seccedaneum Cephalohematoma	Significant head trauma predisposes neonate for development of hyperbilirubinenemia.
Eyes	Placement on face Clear or clouded Drainage	Cloudiness could indicate presence of cataracts. Drainage could be a symptom of inflammation or infection.
Nostrils	Patency (check with #8 French catheter or close off one side at a time with finger and assess for color change)	Inadequate patency could cause respiratory distress. Deviated septum could be cause for inadequate patency.
Mouth	Asymmetry with sucking or crying Palate intact Sucking, rooting, swallowing, gag reflexes	Rules out cleft lip or cleft palate. Deviation or absence could indicate nerve injury or other neurologic problems.
Ears	Normal placement vs. low set	Low-set ears are associated with chromosome abnormalities.

*Note: Gloves should be worn during newborn care until infant is bathed because of concern about potential infection of hospital personnel with blood-borne pathogens such as hepatitis B and AIDS.   *Continued*

IMMEDIATE POSTDELIVERY ASSESSMENT OF THE NEWBORN—continued

	Assessment	Significant Findings
INSPECTION—cont'd		
Chest	Tachypnea, retractions, abdomen for distention	Retractions, tachypnea, and grunting are signs of respiratory distress or difficulty.
Back	Pilonidal dimple or sinus meningomyelocele	Pilonidal dimple or meningomyelocele are central nervous system (CNS) anomalies.
Extremities	Obvious defects or asymmetry of movement Presence or absence of grasp Simian crease Polydactyly or syndactyly	Movement asymmetry or absence of grasp could indicate CNS injury, fracture, or brachial injury. A single palmar crease (Simian) is seen in infants with Down's syndrome.
Skin	Color; staining (meconium), peeling	Staining of skin from meconium indicates previous fetal distress. Dry, peeling, parchment-like skin usually indicates placental dysfunction often due to postmaturity.
Genitalia	Sex determination Ambiguous genitalia	Ambiguous genitalia can indicate genetic problems.

Anus	Present and patent	Meconium passage ensures patency. If not patent, emergency surgery is required.
Cord	Presence of three vessels	A two-vessel cord may be accompanied by other abnormalities.
AUSCULTATION		
Heart	Rate, quality, and location of sounds	If sounds are not heard easily and clearly to left of midline, it could indicate cardiac problems or anomalies. Tachycardia, bradycardia, murmurs, and arrhythmias also indicate possible cardiac dysfunction.
PALPATION		
Chest	Location of maximal heart impulse	Maximum impulse area other than to left of midline could indicate cardiac abnormality.

RAPID ESTIMATION OF GESTATIONAL AGE OF THE NEWBORN

Sites	Gestational Age		
	36 Wk or Less	37-38 Wk	39 Wk or More
Sole creases	Anterior transverse crease only	Occasional creases anterior two thirds	Sole covered with creases
Breast nodule diameter	2 mm	4 mm	7 mm
Scalp hair	Fine and fuzzy	Fine and fuzzy	Coarse and silky
Earlobe	Pliable, no cartilage	Some cartilage	Stiffened by thick cartilage
Testes and scrotum	Testes in lower canal, scrotum small, few rugae	Intermediate	Testes pendulous, scrotum full, extensive rugae

Cunningham FG, MacDonald PC, Gant NF: Williams Obstetrics, 17th ed. Norwalk, Conn, Appleton & Lange, 1989.

FOCUS ASSESSMENT—IMMEDIATE CARE OF NEWBORN

Observe for signs of cyanosis, gagging, nasal flaring, costal breathing, and sternal retractions, respiratory rate less than 60 breaths per minute or more than 30 breaths per minute.

Identify signs of cold stress, e.g., pallor, jitteriness, tremors.

Monitor body temperature.

Observe parent-infant interaction, signs of bonding (e.g., eye contact, cuddling, calling by name).

INTERVENTION

GOALS OF IMMEDIATE CARE

1. Ensure an airway and maintain respirations.
2. Prevent cold stress (hypothermia).
3. Provide a safe environment.
4. Identify actual or potential problems that might require immediate attention.
5. Ensure infant identification.

MECHANICAL SUCTIONING OF NEWBORN

Intervention

1. Attach a #10 French catheter to suction tubing.

2. Turn on suction, place finger over finger-tip control to check negative pressure.

3. Place the end of the catheter into newborn's mouth first (approximately 3 to 5 inches). Place finger over finger-tip control and suction secretions from oropharynx.

Rationale

1. #10 French catheter is correct size for average-sized newborn. Note: If catheter is used to check nasal patency, #8 should be used to prevent trauma to mucous membrane of nares.

2. Negative pressure used is 80 to 100 cm H_2O. Suction should always be checked to be sure that pressure is within this range. (If thick meconium is present, intubation and endotracheal suction are necessary.)

3. No suctioning episode should be greater than 6 seconds so that newborn respiratory depression does not occur.

Continued

MECHANICAL SUCTIONING OF NEWBORN—continued

Intervention	Rationale
4. Rotate suction catheter gently and covering finger-tip control as it is being withdrawn to suction.	4. Prevents trauma to mucous membranes.
5. Suctioning of oropharynx may be repeated if necessary to clear secretions.	5. Note color of infant. Give blow-by oxygen (5L of 100%) if central cyanosis (lips, perioral and mucus membrane) occurs. Repeated suctioning must provide intervals of 10 to 15 seconds recovery time to prevent respiratory depression.
6. Avoid deep suction during early minutes following delivery.	6. Deep suction (suction catheter passing down newborn's throat) can stimulate the vagus nerve causing decrease in heart rate.
7. Do minimum nasopharynx suctioning.	7. Oversuctioning of nares and nasopharynx can traumatize mucous membranes causing edema and respiratory distress.
8. Pass a #8 catheter into nasopharynx to determine patency.	8. Newborns are obligatory nasal breathers so patency should be determined. Larger catheter may cause trauma.
9. After the initial minutes following delivery, some primary health care givers pass a suction catheter through the mouth into the stomach to empty gastric contents.	9. Suctioning episode should not be greater than 6 seconds. Gastric contents that are acidic are removed to prevent aspiration, which could cause a chemical pneumonitis.

CONTROLLING MECHANISMS OF HEAT LOSS

Mechanisms of Heat Loss

Evaporation: Loss of heat when water on the skin is converted to vapor

Conduction: Loss of heat to a cooler surface (unwarmed bed, cool scale, cold stethoscope, cold hands) by direct skin contact

Convection: Loss of heat from warm body surface to cooler air currents such as air-conditioned rooms, unwarmed oxygen, or not using radiant warmer for care

Radiation: Loss of heat from body surfaces to cooler surfaces and objects not in direct contact with the body, (e.g., walls of a room or window)

Preventing Heat Loss

First step in newborn care is to immediately dry infant and remove wet linen.

Place on prewarmed bed under radiant heat source for care. Cover scale with blanket before weighing infant, warm bell of stethoscope in hands before auscultating infant's chest, and warm hands before handling neonate (rub together under warm water).

Check placement of warmed bed or radiant warmer to ensure the area is free from drafts and is away from air vents. Use warmed humified oxygen if needed for oxygenation and keep newborn wrapped when not skin-to-skin or under radiant warmer with temperature probe attached.

Use temperature probe to help maintain stable skin temperature, avoid placing warmed bed or radiant warmer next to outside wall or windows that are not well insulated. Turn up thermostat in room prior to delivery.

CONSEQUENCE OF COLD STRESS (HYPOTHERMIA)

1. Hypoglycemia: Metabolism increases to maintain or produce heat, which depletes glycogen stores.
2. Hypoxia: O_2 consumption increases to produce more body heat, which can lead to metabolic acidosis due to anaerobic metabolism.
3. Inhibition of surfactant production: Creates potential for development of severe respiratory distress.

SIGNS OF HYPOTHERMIA IN THE NEWBORN

1. Skin feels cool to touch
2. Acrocyanosis (hands and feet are blue) or mottling of skin particularly in extremities due to vasoconstriction; may become centrally cyanotic
3. Quiet, less responsive
4. Jitteriness possibly indicative of hypoglycemia
5. Increased respiratory rate (tachypnea) and development of respiratory distress and acidosis

NURSING PROCEDURE: EYE PROPHYLAXIS

Intervention

1. Lay out tube of erythromycin ophthalmic ointment and sterile cotton balls. Note: Do not place under radiant warmer.

2. Gently clean the skin around the eyes with sterile cotton (cotton may be moistened with sterile water).

3. Using the first finger and thumb (in the same position as holding a pencil) gently open the infant's eyelids.

4. Instill a thin line of ointment (at least ½ inch or 1 to 2 cm) along the lower conjunctival area from the inner aspect of the eye outward. (Be careful not to touch another part of the eye with the tube.)

5. Carefully manipulate lids to spread and distribute ointment.

6. After about 1 minute, gently wipe off any excess ointment from eyelids and surrounding skin with sterile cotton ball. (May be moistened with sterile water.)

Rationale

1. To have available for eye prophylaxis. Infection control principle is that each infant will have his own ointment and cotton balls.

2. Clears debris of blood and vernix away from eyes and provides traction for the fingers when gently opening the eye to instill the ointment.

3. This must be done gently to minimize trauma to the soft tissues around the eye.

4. The normal lubrication of the eye will distribute the ointment. Touching the eye with the tube could cause trauma and be a source of infection.

5. This should also be done gently to assist spread of ointment and prevent trauma.

6. Do not irrigate the eye after instillation because it may wash away the effectiveness of the prophylaxis.

SUMMARY OF POSTDELIVERY CARE OF THE NEONATE

1. Wash hands and don gloves.
2. Note time of delivery.
3. Receive newborn in warmed blankets and place under radiant warmer. Dry briefly and discard wet blankets.
4. Attach temperature probe (tape in place) to newborn's abdomen. Set temperature set point at 36 to 36.5°C.
5. Briefly suction oropharyngeal to ensure patent airway. Nasopharynx can be suctioned or each nostril can be blocked one at a time to assess patency.
6. Complete 1-minute Apgar.
7. Blow-by oxygen may be given for central cyanosis.
8. Check capillary refill time. Blanche skin over chest and assess how quickly the blood returns.
9. Assess respirations and auscultate chest for heart and breath sounds.
10. Complete the 5-minute Apgar score.
11. Count number of cord vessels present.
12. Evaluate for obvious gross abnormalities of infant.
13. Place identification bracelets and security disc on wrists or ankles.
14. Administer vitamin K (phytonadione) 0.5 to 1 mg IM. May be given in the delivery area or after admitted to nursery.
15. Place erythromycin ophthalmic ointment in each eye. May be done in the delivery area or after admitted to nursery.
16. Wipe off newborn's feet and footprint.
17. Wrap infant and give to parents to hold.
18. Assess and record parent's initial reaction and responses to the newborn.
19. Assist mother to breast-feed if she desires.
20. Evaluate infant's respirations, color, heart rate, and temperature and note any changes that are indicative of problems.
21. Document all care.

TRANSFERRING NEWBORN TO NURSERY CARE

1. The newborn is transported to the nursery in the mother's arms or in a baby bed.
2. On arrival in the nursery both the transferring labor and delivery nurse and the receiving nursery nurse

   a. Check the identification bracelets to verify name and identification number with information noted in the chart
   b. Verify the sex of the newborn
   c. Verify the official newborn's weight
3. The newborn is placed under a radiant warmer.
4. The following report information is communicated by the transferring labor and delivery nurse to the receiving nursery nurse:
   a. Maternal prenatal history
      (1) Last menstrual period and expected date of confinement
      (2) Medical or obstetric complications
   b. Maternal blood type and Rh factor
      (1) Tests done if mother is Rh negative
   c. Maternal screening for infection
      (1) Rubella titer
      (2) VDRL
      (3) Herpes
   d. Labor history
      (1) Onset and length of labor
      (2) When membranes ruptured
      (3) Nature of amniotic fluid
      (4) Medications received by mother
      (5) Anesthesia used during labor and delivery
   e. Fetal monitor tracing
   f. Delivery information
      (1) Length of second stage
      (2) Medications administered in delivery room
      (3) Type of delivery
      (4) Operative obstetric procedures used
   g. Post delivery care
      (1) Apgar score
      (2) If resuscitation was required, medications administered
      (3) Evidence of birth injury
      (4) Passage of urine or stool
      (5) Parent-infant interaction
      (6) If newborn was breast-fed

NURSING CARE PLAN

IMMEDIATE CARE OF THE NEWBORN

Goals (expected outcomes)	Interventions	Rationale	Evaluation
INEFFECTIVE THERMOREGULATION—RELATED TO EXTREME SUDDEN CHANGE IN ENVIRONMENTAL TEMPERATURE AND NEWBORN STATUS			
Infant will maintain normal temperature.	Wrap infant in warmed blankets or place on warmed bed (if given to mother for skin-to-skin contact place warmed blankets over mother and infant).	Minimizes heat loss by conduction, convection, and radiation.	Infant's temperature is 97.7 to 98.6°F (axillary) or 97.8 to 99°F (rectally).
	Dry briefly and quickly discard wet linens. Apply warm, dry blankets. Put a hat on infant's head. (Some hospitals place the infant in a plastic bag that comes up under the arms.)	Minimizes or prevents unnecessary evaporative loss. Heat loss increases metabolism and O_2 consumption.	

Continued

NURSING CARE PLAN

IMMEDIATE CARE OF THE NEWBORN—continued

Goals (expected outcomes)	Interventions	Rationale	Evaluation
INEFFECTIVE THERMOREGULATION—RELATED TO EXTREME SUDDEN CHANGE IN ENVIRONMENTAL TEMPERATURE AND NEWBORN STATUS—cont'd			
	If on heated bed, attach temperature probe to abdomen about midway between umbilicus and lower border of the sternum.	Monitors body temperature.	Infant maintains skin temperature at 97.7 to 98.6°F.
INEFFECTIVE AIRWAY CLEARANCE—RELATED TO OROPHARYNGEAL SECRETIONS			
Infant will begin to breathe and cry lustily.	Mouth and then nose suctioned with bulb syringe when head delivered.	Removes oropharyngeal secretions. Mouth always suctioned first. When nares are suctioned it could cause a reflex gasp, causing possibility of aspiration.	Newborn requires minimal suctioning and establishes respiratory activity.
	Place infant on radiant warmer in supine position with neck slightly extended (so that neck is straight).	Ensures patent airway.	Newborn exhibits 40 to 60 unlabored respirations per minute.

Goal	Interventions	Rationale	Outcome
	nose (with bulb, mechanical or DeLee) if needed. Initiate tracheal suctioning if meconium present.	...sures patent airway. Clears airway to prevent meconium aspiration or pneumonia.	Lungs are clear to auscultation. Newborn exhibits no signs of respiratory distress.

INEFFECTIVE BREATHING PATTERNS—RELATED TO INTRAPARTUM HYPOXIA

Goal	Interventions	Rationale	Outcome
Newborn will establish successful gas exchange with regular pattern of breathing at respiratory rate of 40 to 60.	Provide brief stimulation to initiate respirations if necessary (rub back twice or flick soles twice—no more).	Stimulates breathing.	Newborn spontaneously initiates regular pattern of breathing at respiratory rate of 40 to 60.
	Initiate resuscitation if still not breathing—positive pressure ventilation with 100% oxygen at 5L with bag and mask for 30 seconds and then reevaluate respirations, then heart rate and then color.	Initiates respirations, maintains oxygenation to prevent further hypoxic depression.	Newborn responds to resuscitation. Establishes normal newborn breathing pattern.
	Initiate tracheal suctioning if meconium present.	Clears airway so breathing occurs and hypoxia and aspiration prevented.	Newborn is breathing freely; color is pink; and is active and responsive.
	Auscultate breathing sounds.	Determines need for further suctioning.	Normal breath sounds auscultated.

Continued

NURSING CARE PLAN

IMMEDIATE CARE OF THE NEWBORN—continued

Goals (expected outcomes)	Interventions	Rationale	Evaluation
ALTERED TISSUE PERFUSION—RELATED TO HYPOTHERMIA			
Color will be pink by time of 1-minute Apgar score (some acrocyanosis may be present).	Place on warm bed, dry, remove wet linen, wrap in warm blankets, and place hat on head.	Prevents heat loss.	Apgar score of 7 to 10 at 1 and 5 minutes of age. Temperature 97.7 to 98.8°F. Apical pulse 120 to 160. Infant exhibits rapid capillary refill.
	Administer 5L of free flow oxygen if infant exhibits central cyanosis.	Ensures breathing is satisfactory rate of 40 to 60 and heart rate is greater than 100. Assess perfusion. Ensures no cold stress. Ensures adequate oxygenation and perfusion.	
POTENTIAL FOR INFECTION—RELATED TO IMMATURITY OF IMMUNE SYSTEM			
Normal infection-free infant will leave hospital.	Wash hands and apply gloves to prepare for initial care.	Universal precautions for self-protection from body fluids and secretions.	Infant displays no signs or symptoms of infection.

Ask all who will observe delivery to wash hands and wear a gown.	Ensures infection control and maintains cleanliness. Some hospitals do not require gowning but do ask all observers to wash their hands prior to handling or touching the infant.	Infant has no trauma of the eyes and is free of conjunctivitis and eye infection.
Gently open eyes and apply prophylactic erythromycin eye ointment.	Minimizes trauma to soft tissues around the eyes. Antibiotic ointment prevents ophthalmia neonatorium, chlamydia, and other infections.	

ALTERED PARENTING—RELATED TO RECENT BIRTH OF INFANT

Family is excited about being together.		
Encourage family interaction before, during, and after birth.	Encourages family attachment in atmosphere of openness just after birth. Nurse can assist with getting reciprocal interactions to occur between parents and infant.	Family interacts spontaneously and favorably.

Continued

NURSING CARE PLAN

IMMEDIATE CARE OF THE NEWBORN—continued

Goals (expected outcomes)	Interventions	Rationale	Evaluation
ALTERED PARENTING—RELATED TO RECENT BIRTH OF INFANT—cont'd			
	Allow couple to hold and get to know newborn as soon as possible after birth.	Bonding occurs from conception through birth and beyond, but immediately after birth is a sensitive period for attaching and additional bonding.	
	Point out features and try to make the first interaction as positive as possible.	If the infant responds in a positive way, it causes a positive response from the parents and reciprocal relationship gives a boost to the process of attaching.	
KNOWLEDGE DEFICIT—RELATED TO CARE AND BEHAVIOR OF THE NEWBORN			
Family has positive attitude about their birth experience and are	Promote rooming in (if available). Point out reflexes, how to	Every interaction the nurse has with the family should include as much	Family can verbalize how to use resources and knows to ask the nurse or physi-

comfortable about asking questions.	get infant to open eyes by tilting back and then upright.	teaching as they can handle at a time. Again this enhances the attachment process.	cian if they have questions.
	Describe some of the obvious characteristics.	Pointing out characteristics helps the couple to learn about their infant and enhance attachment.	Infant is quiet, alert, looking around, and responsive to parents.
	Assist the mother to breast-feed in the delivery area if she has decided to breast-feed.	After delivery most newborns are in an alert state and ready to suck and breast-feed.	Infant goes to breast eagerly, and mother and infant have a successful new experience. Colostrum is very nutritious.
	Encourage couple to talk to infant.	Talking, stroking, making eye contact are a part of "falling in love" with their infant and the infant is capable of responding.	Parents and infant enjoy a reciprocal getting acquainted period.
	Describe resources available for teaching— videos, booklets, phone numbers.	Couple can be introduced to teaching that is and will be available to assist them in their parenting role.	Parents are asking questions about resources for learning about parenting.

Chapter 11

NEWBORN ASSESSMENT AND ONGOING CARE

This chapter focuses on nursing care of the newborn and supportive actions that assist the infant to adapt successfully to extrauterine life.

LABORATORY VALUES

EXPECTED VALUES FOR FULL-TERM INANT

RBC count	5,000,000-7,000,000/µl
Hemoglobin	14-20 g/dl
Hematocrit	55%
Blood glucose	45-97 mg/dl
Calcium	7.3-9.2 mmg/dl

SIGNS OF DANGER TO THE NEWBORN

Parents should promptly report the occurrence of any of the following to the primary health care provider:

- Skin color changes: cyanosis around the mouth (circumoral), jaundice
- Periods of apnea lasting longer than 15 sec
- Any change in feeding patterns, i.e., more than one episode of refusing to nurse or feed from the bottle
- Repeated emesis or episodes of projectile vomiting after feeding
- Bleeding from the umbilical cord stump area or circumcision
- Any signs of infection:
  a. Rectal temperature >101°F (38.4°C) or <97°F (36.1°C)
  b. Eye redness, swelling, or discharge
  c. Redness, swelling, or discharge from the umbilical cord stump area
  d. Excessive crying or fussiness, lethargy, or difficulty in rousing the infant
  e. Two or more green, watery stools, flatus, and irritability
- Any change in elimination patterns that persists longer than 12 hr, e.g., loose stools or hard, packed stools, decline in number of wet diapers to less than five to eight

SUMMARY OF NEWBORN PHYSICAL ASSESSMENT

Assessment area	Usual findings	Deviations
GENERAL OBSERVATIONS		
Muscle tone	Flexed position; good tone	"Floppy"; rigid or tense
Skin		
Color	Pink tone to ruddy when crying; appropriate to ethnic origin; acrocyanosis	Pallor; cyanosis; jaundice; ecchymosis; petechiae
Texture	Smooth; dryness with some peeling; lanugo on back; vernix	Excessive peeling or cracking; roughness
Rashes and pigmentation	Erythema toxicum; milia; mongolian spots	Impetigo; hemangiomas; nevus flammeus (port-wine stain)
Hydration	Skin pinch over abdomen immediately returns to original state	Skin maintains "tent" shape after pinch
Cry	Lusty	Shrill; weak; grunty
MEASUREMENTS		
Weight	2700-4000 g (6-9 lb)	
Length	48-53 cm (19-21 in)	
Head circumference	33-37 cm (13-14½ in)	
Chest circumference	31-35 cm (12-14 in)	

Continued

SUMMARY OF NEWBORN PHYSICAL ASSESSMENT—continued

Assessment area	Usual findings	Deviations
VITAL SIGNS		
Temperature	Axillary (preferred method): 36.5°-37°C (97.7°-98.6°F) Rectal: 36.5°-37.2°C (97.7°-99°F)	Hypothermia; fever
Respirations	40-60 respirations/min; quiet and shallow; diaphragmatic; occasional periods of rapid breathing, alternating with short periods of apnea	Prolonged rapid breathing; apnea lasting longer than 10 sec; grunting; retractions; persistent slow rate
Heart rate (apical pulse)	120-160 beats/min; faster when crying (up to 180 beats/min); slower when sleeping (down to 100 beats/min)	Tachycardia: >160 beats/min at rest Bradycardia: <120 beats/min when awake
HEAD	Vaginal delivery: elongated (molding) Breech or cesarean birth: round, sym- metric Size within normal range	Caput succedaneum; cephalohematoma; hydrocephaly; microcephaly
FONTANELS		
Anterior	Flat; soft; firm Diamond shaped; 2-3 cm wide; 3-4 cm long; smaller at birth with molding	Bulging; sunken Small; almost closed; closed (craniostenosis); widened
Posterior	Triangular shape; small; almost closed	Enlarged
FACE	Small; round; symmetric; fat pads in cheeks; receding chin	Asymmetric; distorted
Eyes	Edematous lids; usually closed; blue or slate	Elevation or ptosis of lids; epicanthal folds;

	Normal	Abnormal
	gray color; no tears; red reflex present; pupils equal, round, react to light Common variations: subconjunctival hemorrhages; chemical conjunctivitis; occasional slight nystagmus or convergent strabismus	absence of red reflex; unequal, dilated, or constricted pupils Purulent discharge; frequent nystagmus; constant, divergent, or unilateral strabismus
Mouth	Intact lips, gums, palate; epithelial pearls; "sucking blisters" on lips; tongue midline, mobile, appropriate size for mouth, can extend to alveolar ridge	Cleft lip or palate; white, cheesy patches on tongue, gums, or mucous membrane; large or protruding tongue
Nose	In midline; even placement in relation to eyes and mouth; nares patent; septum intact, midline	Flattened or bruised; unusual placement or configuration; obstructed nares; deviated or perforated septum
Ears	Well-formed cartilage; appropriate size for head; upper attachment on line extended through inner and outer canthus of eye; external auditory canal patent	Floppy, large and protruding; malformed; low set; obstruction of canal
NECK	Short; thick; full range of motion; no masses	Webbing; abnormal shortening; limitation of motion; torticollis; masses
Clavicles	Straight; smooth; intact	Knot or lump; decreased movement of extremity on one side
THORAX	Round; symmetric; protruding xiphoid process	Assymmetric; funnel chest
Breath sounds	Loud; bronchial; bilaterally equal	Decreased breath sounds; increased breath sounds

Continued

SUMMARY OF NEWBORN PHYSICAL ASSESSMENT—continued

Assessment area	Usual findings	Deviations
THORAX—cont'd		
Heart sounds	Regular rate and rhythm; first and second sounds clear and distinct	Murmurs; dysrhythmias
Breasts	Symmetric; flat with erect nipples; engorgement second or third day not unusual	Redness and firmness around nipple
ABDOMEN	Symmetric; slightly protuberant; no masses	Scaphoid or concave shape; distention; palpable masses
Liver	Palpable 2-3 cm below right costal margin	Enlargement
Spleen	Tip may be palpable in left upper quadrant	Enlargement
Kidneys	May be palpable at level of umbilicus	Enlargement
Femoral pulses	Bilaterally equal	Unequal or absent
Umbilicus	No extensive protrusion or herniation; no signs of infection	Umbilical hernia; omphalocele; redness; induration; foul-smelling discharge
	Cord: bluish white, moist → black, dry; three vessels; no oozing or bleeding	Two vessels; bleeding or oozing from stump
GENITALIA	Appropriate for gender	Ambiguous genitalia
Female		
Labia	Edematous; labia majora cover labia minora; vernix in creases	Hematoma; lesions; fusion of labia
Vagina	Mucus discharge, possibly blood tinged	

Male		
Foreskin	Adherent to glans penis	Opening below tip of penis (hypospadias)
Urethra	Opening at tip of penis	Opening above tip of penis (epispadias)
Testes	Palpable in each scrotal sac	Palpable in inguinal canal; not palpable
POSTERIOR OF BODY		
Spinal column	Straight, flexible; intact; no masses	Exaggerated curves; spina bifida; any masses; pilonidal cyst
Anus	Patent	Imperforate anus, anal fissures
Extremities	Symmetric in size, shape, and movement	Unequal or abnormal size or shape; asymmetric or limited movement of one or more extremities
Digits	Five on each hand and foot; appropriate size and shape	Missing digits; syndactyly (webbing); polydactyly (extra digits)
Hips	Even leg length, knee height, gluteal folds; no resistance or limitation to abduction	Uneven leg length, knee height, or gluteal folds; uneven or limited abduction; hip "click" or "clunk" on abduction
Feet	Straight, or postural deviation easily corrected with gentle pressure	Structural deformities: talipes equinovarus (clubfoot); metatarsus adductus

Continued

SUMMARY OF NEWBORN PHYSICAL ASSESSMENT—continued

Assessment area	Usual findings	Deviations
REFLEXES		
Rooting and sucking	Turns toward object touching cheek, lips, or corner of mouth; opens mouth; begins sucking movements; strong suck, pulls object into mouth	No rooting; weak ineffective, or absent suck
	May be diminished or absent after eating	
Grasp		
Palmar	Fingers grasp object when palm stimulated and hang on briefly	Weak or absent
Plantar	Toes curl downward when soles of feet are stimulated	Weak or absent
Moro	Symmetric response to sudden stimulus: lateral extension of arms with opening of hands, followed by flexion and adduction	Asymmetric; absent; incomplete
Stepping	Stepping movements when infant held upright with sole of foot touching surface	Asymmetric or absent

NURSING PROCEDURE: HEEL STICK FOR BLOOD GLUCOSE

Intervention	Rationale
1. Warm infant's heel by wrapping foot in warm, moist compress for 3 to 5 min.	1. Increases circulation.
2. Cleanse heel with alcohol.	2. Minimizes risk of infection from puncture.
3. Allow to dry.	3. Reduces potential for hemolysis or tissue irritation.
4. Identify site on lateral aspect of heel.	4. Avoids accidental puncture of medial plantar artery or injury to nerves.
5. Rapidly puncture heel with sterile disposable lancet.	5. Minimizes trauma.
6. Remove first drop of blood with sterile gauze.	6. Reduces potential for dilution with tissue fluid.
7. Collect generous sample of blood on test strip. Avoid squeezing foot.	7. Squeezing foot may dilute blood sample with tissue fluid.
8. If using Dextrostix: wait 60 sec before rinsing off blood under steady stream of water.	8. Ensures accurate reading.
9. If using glucometer (e.g., Acucheck): immediately press timer button. At exactly 60 sec lightly wipe off all blood with a clean, dry cotton ball.	9. Ensures accurate reading.
10. Place test strip in meter slot before timer reaches 120 sec.	10. Reading will appear in display window after 120 sec.
11. Apply adhesive bandage to puncture site while waiting.	11. Protects from infection and further trauma.
12. Record results.	12. Enables comparison with preceding and later tests.

CLIENT SELF-CARE EDUCATION: CARE OF THE UMBILICAL CORD STUMP

Action	**Rationale**
1. Fold and anchor top of diaper below level of cord stump.	1. Avoids irritation and allows air circulation to hasten drying.
2. Use a cotton ball and 70% alcohol to cleanse area between stump and skin. This should be done two to three times daily or with each diaper change. Continue until cord has detached and umbilicus has healed completely.	2. Hastens drying and sloughing of remainder of cord stump.
3. Avoid use of tub baths until umbilical area has healed completely.	3. Further hastens drying; reduces potential for injury.
4. Avoid dislodging cord before it heals completely.	4. May cause bleeding. Cord usually falls off between day 5 and day 14 after birth.
5. Promptly report any signs of bleeding, inflammation, or discharge from area around stump.	5. May indicate injury or infection and should be evaluated by primary health provider.

CLIENT SELF-CARE EDUCATION: CIRCUMCISION CARE

Action

1a. Observe for bleeding at every diaper change.

  b. Report any evidence of bleeding immediately.

2. Plastibell is left in place. Do not attempt to remove.

3. If petroleum gauze has been applied, leave in place unless soiled by urine or stool. A petroleum dressing usually is used for 24 to 48 hours.

4. Monitor voiding for size of stream, amount of urine, and bloody urine.

5. When changing the diaper, hold infant's ankles with one hand.

6. At each diaper change place infant in position for inspection of penis.
Squeeze a gentle cascade of warm water over penis.

7. Fasten diaper loosely for first 48 hours after circumcision.

8. Yellowish-white exudate may be noted for 2 to 3 days. Do not remove this exudate.

9. During daily bath follow procedure outlined in No. 6. Use warm soapy water for initial cascade. Rinse well with warm water cascades and pat dry.

10. Report promptly any sign of ulceration or difficulty voiding before or after discharge home.

Rationale

1a. Although rare, bleeding is a potential complication of circumcision.

  b. Enables prompt treatment.

2. Does not interfere with voiding or healing. Usually falls off within 3 to 4 days.

3. Protects the surgical site from irritation. Soiling increases potential for irritation and infection.

4. Although rare, damage to urethra is one potential postoperative complication.

5. Prevents infant from kicking against operative site.

6. Facilitates adequate visualization of penis.

Rinses away urine; reduces potential for irritation.

7. Avoids pressure on the operative area. Reduces discomfort.

8. Signals normal granulation and healing.

9. Cleanses, promotes healing and comfort.

10. Requires evaluation by primary health care provider.

NURSING CARE PLAN

ONGOING CARE OF THE HEALTHY NEWBORN

INEFFECTIVE THERMOREGULATION—RELATED TO LIMITED METABOLIC ABILITY TO COMPENSATE FOR CHANGES IN ENVIRONMENTAL TEMPERATURE

Goals (expected outcomes)	Interventions	Rationale	Evaluation
Infant will experience uneventful thermal adaptation to extrauterine life.	Maintain environmental temperature of 72° to 76°F (22° to 26°C).	Ensures thermal neutrality. Reduces potential for hyperthermia or hypothermia (minimizes energy expenditure).	Infant's vital signs remain within acceptable range (see previous discussion).
	Avoid placing infant on cold surfaces.	Minimizes heat loss through conduction.	
	Keep infant dry, warm and covered.	Minimizes heat loss through evaporation, radiation, and convection.	
	Dress in shirt and diaper; wrap in warm blanket; cover with blanket; place cap on head for transport.		
	Avoid placing infant in drafts, near cold walls, or windows.	Minimizes heat loss through evaporation, radiation, and convection.	

Minimize exposure during infant care, e.g., bath.	Protects from air currents.	Infant exhibits no signs of hyperthermia or hypothermia.
Transport to mother in crib.	Protects from air currents.	
Client teaching:		
Explain importance of maintaining thermal neutrality to parents.	Enables parents to understand reasons for dressing infant to minimize environmental stress.	
Discuss methods of preventing overheating and chilling (see above).	Enables parents to protect newborn from environmental stressors.	
Describe signs of heat and cold stress.	Facilitates early identification of thermal stress.	
Discuss immediate treatment:	Enables parents to intervene appropriately to minimize consequences.	
Cold stress—cover, wrap, cuddle.		
Heat stress—remove coverings; sponge with tepid water.		
Demonstrate method of taking axillary temperature.	Enables parents to gather assessment data required.	Parents take and read axillary temperature accurately.

Continued

NURSING CARE PLAN

ONGOING CARE OF THE HEALTHY NEWBORN—continued

Goals (expected outcomes)	Interventions	Rationale	Evaluation
INEFFECTIVE THERMOREGULATION—RELATED TO LIMITED METABOLIC ABILITY TO COMPENSATE FOR CHANGES IN ENVIRONMENTAL TEMPERATURE—cont'd			
	Emphasize importance of reporting significant changes in infant status and behaviors promptly.	Facilitates prompt and definitive nursing and medical management.	After discharge, parents report elevated or subnormal temperatures promptly to primary health care provider.
POTENTIAL FOR ASPIRATION/INEFFECTIVE AIRWAY CLEARANCE—RELATED TO EXCESSIVE OROPHARYNGEAL MUCUS			
Infant will experience unimpaired gas exchange.	Support newborn in side-lying position with rolled blanket from shoulders to rump.	Facilitates drainage.	Infant's respiratory rate is 30-50 per minute.
	Suction mouth and nostrils gently with bulb syringe as needed to remove excess mucus.	Maintains patent airway; reduces risk of aspiration.	Infant has no evidence of nasal flaring, sternal retractions, grunting, or gagging.
	Position infant on right side after feeding.	Encourages escape of air from stomach.	
	Avoid placing unattended infant in supine position.	Minimizes risk of mucus' occluding oropharynx.	

Withhold feeding immediately before circumcision.

Client teaching:

Explain rationale for specific infant positioning and avoiding placing child in supine position while unattended.

Demonstrate proper use of the bulb syringe.

Minimizes risk of regurgitation and aspiration while in supine position.

Minimizes risk of aspiration.

Enables parents to take prompt action if needed.

Parents verbalize understanding signs of respiratory distress; respond accurately to questions.

Parents demonstrate appropriate infant positioning.

Parents demonstrate suctioning with bulb syringe.

Parents verbalize confidence in own ability to perform procedure safely and effectively.

Continued

NURSING CARE PLAN

ONGOING CARE OF THE HEALTHY NEWBORN—continued

Goals (expected outcomes)	Interventions	Rationale	Evaluation
POTENTIAL FOR INFECTION—RELATED TO IMMATURE IMMUNE SYSTEM			
Infant will experience minimum exposure to potential pathogens.	Maintain good handwashing technique. Wash hands before and after providing care.	Minimizes risk of transmitting microorganisms from self, environment, or from infant to infant.	Infant's vital signs remain within normal range. Infant is active; responsive; feeds well. Chemical conjunctivitis (if present from eye Credé maneuver) subsides in 3 to 4 days; infant exhibits no purulent drainage from eyes.
—RELATED TO IMPAIRED SKIN INTEGRITY SECONDARY TO UMBILICAL CORD STUMP			
Infant will remain free of infection.	Apply alcohol to umbilical cord stump with every diaper change. Apply bactericidal preparation to stump as ordered.	Hastens drying of cord, closing potential portal of entry. Antibiotic ointment or Triple dye reduces risk of infection.	Exhibits no signs of local infection (redness, swelling, drainage) in area of umbilical stump (or circumcision site if applicable).

—RELATED TO IMPAIRED SKIN INTEGRITY SECONDARY TO CIRCUMCISION

Infant will remain free of infection.	Minimize potential for irritation or contamination of circumcision site.	
	Apply diaper loosely; place infant in side-lying position.	Minimizes irritation from pressure and friction.
	Change diapers often; cleanse area with warm water cascade; change petroleum gauze if soiled with urine or stool.	Minimizes irritation from urine or stool.
		Discourages growth of bacterial contaminants.
	Record and report any signs of infection promptly.	Enables prompt and definitive management.
	Client teaching:	
	Discuss and demonstrate methods of preventing infection:	Enables parents to minimize infant's exposure to potential pathogens.
	Handwashing	
	Preventing contact with contaminated surfaces	
Healing progresses without interruption.		
Parents verbalize understanding of basic principles of infection control		
Parents demonstrate appropriate handwashing technique.		

Continued

NURSING CARE PLAN

ONGOING CARE OF THE HEALTHY NEWBORN—continued

Goals (expected outcomes)	Interventions	Rationale	Evaluation
—RELATED TO IMPAIRED SKIN INTEGRITY SECONDARY TO CIRCUMCISION—cont'd			
	Avoiding contact with persons who are not well		
	Use of masks		
	Cord care		Parents demonstrate appropriate care of umbilical cord stump.
	Care of circumcision		Parents demonstrate appropriate care of circumcision.
	Describe signs of infection.	Facilitates early identification.	
	Instruct parent to record and report any signs of infection promptly to health care provider.	Enables prompt and definitive medical management.	After discharge parents promptly report any signs of deviations from expected progress to primary health care provider.

POTENTIAL FLUID VOLUME DEFICIT—RELATED TO MARGINAL COAGULABILITY SECONDARY TO LACK OF NECESSARY INTESTINAL FLORA AND CIRCUMCISION

Infant will experience uneventful postoperative course.	Administer prophylactic vitamin K injection as ordered.	Provides cofactor required for transformation of prothrombin precursor to active prothrombin.
		Infant exhibits no evidence of bleeding.
		Infant heals without incident.
	Avoid pressure, friction, or injury of circumcision site.	Reduces potential for traumatic bleeding.
	Cover site with petroleum gauze as ordered; remove only when soiled. Cleanse area with warm water cascade.	Minimizes trauma to delicate tissue.
	Record and report bleeding to primary health provider promptly.	Enables prompt and definitive treatment.
	In the event of bleeding, apply oxidizing cellulose gauze (Oxycel) as ordered.	Enhances clotting.
	Client teaching:	
	Discuss the appropriate management of circumcision.	Enables client understanding.
		Parents demonstrate safe, effective care of circumcision site.

Continued

NURSING CARE PLAN

ONGOING CARE OF THE HEALTHY NEWBORN—continued

Goals (expected outcomes)	Interventions	Rationale	Evaluation
POTENTIAL FLUID VOLUME DEFICIT—RELATED TO MARGINAL COAGULABILITY SECONDARY TO LACK OF NECESSARY INTESTINAL FLORA AND CIRCUMCISION—cont'd			
	Explain rationale for actions.	Increases potential for client compliance with behaviors recommended.	
	Demonstrate cleansing of circumcision site (see Client Self-Care Education: Circumcision Care).	Enables parents to participate actively in infant's care; continues safe care after discharge.	
	Describe signs of complications (e.g., bleeding, changes in urinary elimination pattern).	Facilitates early identification and prompt management of problems.	
	Demonstrate assessment of infant hydration status.	Facilitates early identification and prompt management of problems.	
	Instruct parents to report any signs of deviation from expected behaviors.	Enables prompt and definitive management of problems.	

ALTERED NUTRITION: LESS THAN BODY REQUIREMENTS—RELATED TO LIMITED INTAKE, HYPOGLYCEMIA

Infant will exhibit normal fluid and electrolyte balance.	Begin feedings in accordance with protocol or primary health provider's orders.	Newborn has a high metabolic rate; requires glucose to meet energy needs.	Infant feeds well; is active; has lusty cry.
			Infant exhibits no signs of hypoglycemia (jittery; tremors; irregular respirations, apnea; pallor; cyanosis.
			Infant has capillary blood glucose level: >45 mg/dl
	First feeding: 15 ml 5% glucose in water.	Water is easily and rapidly absorbed; glucose is rapidly available to meet needs.	
	Offer feedings every 3 to 4 hr or on demand (breast or formula).		Infant exhibits weight loss of less than 10% of birth weight during first 3 to 4 days after birth.
	Burp infant frequently during feedings.	Encourages expulsion of air swallowed during feeding; reduces risk of regurgitation.	
	Place infant on right side after feeding.	Facilitates escape of air from stomach; reduces risk of regurgitation.	Infant exhibits no regurgitation of feedings.

Continued

NURSING CARE PLAN

ONGOING CARE OF THE HEALTHY NEWBORN—continued

Goals (expected outcomes)	Interventions	Rationale	Evaluation
ALTERED NUTRITION: LESS THAN BODY REQUIREMENTS—RELATED TO LIMITED INTAKE, HYPOGLYCEMIA—cont'd			
	Client teaching: Explain rationale for current nursing management.	Enables parental understanding; reduces anxiety.	
	Demonstrate techniques for burping, positioning.	Allows parents to participate actively in infant care; reduces potential for regurgitation.	
EFFECTIVE PARENTING			
Mother or parents will gain information and skills needed to provide safe, effective infant care; exhibit growing competence and confidence in providing infant care;	Target teaching to specific individual knowledge deficits (see preceding information and specific Client Self-Care Education).	Maximizes parental knowledge gain.	Parents actively participate in own learning.

and provide safe, effective care appropriate to infant's specific needs.	Demonstrate necessary actions and explain rationale.	Enables parental understanding of need for specific actions; facilitates compliance with nursing recommendations.	Parents seek information and guidance to meet individual learning needs.
	Invite and answer questions as they arise.	Identifies additional learning needs.	Parents verbalize beginning confidence in their knowledge base.
	Provide guidance as needed by parents during return-demonstrations.	Supports parents' growing competence and self-confidence.	Parents demonstrate increasing confidence in ability to provide safe, effective newborn care.
			Parents perform procedures safely and accurately.
			Infant progresses normally without occurrence of common complications of the neonatal period.
			Vital signs stable within normal limits
			Alert, responsive
			Feeds well
			Maintains normal weight gain

Chapter   12

INFANT NUTRITION

CHOICE OF FEEDING METHOD

Choosing the method for feeding is an important and sometimes difficult decision for parents to make. Their choice is influenced by a variety of factors such as personal attitudes, their culture, social pressures, and psychologic needs of the mother.

Information about the differences in available feeding methods can be useful in helping parents make a decision based on facts. Even though the health professional believes breast-feeding is ideal, care must be taken not to force the mother to choose this method, and the mother who chooses to bottle-feed should not be made to feel guilty. Once the feeding method has been chosen, the nurse should focus on providing support to ensure the chosen method is successful.

ADVANTAGES OF BREAST-FEEDING

Breast milk contains ideal nutrients needed for optimum growth of the human neonate.

Breast milk protects the infant against diarrhea. Intestinal flora of the breast-fed infant produces feces with a pH of 5 to 6. This low pH inhibits the growth of bacteria such as *Escherichia coli,* which can cause diarrhea in the infant.

The incidence of respiratory infections is lower in breast-fed infants.

Proteins found in human milk are almost nonallergenic to human infants. The incidence of allergic diseases is lower in breast-fed infants with a family history of allergies.

Breast-feeding promotes uterine involution in the mother, and oxytocin is released when the infant sucks.

Breast milk is readily available at the right temperature.

ASSESSMENT

BREAST-FEEDING

1. Assess the mother's ability to assume a comfortable position.
2. Assess mother's nipples for the following:
   a. Pliability   d. Abrasions
   b. Inversion   e. Tenderness
   c. Cracks   f. Pain
3. Assess breasts for the following:
   a. Engorgement
   b. Plugged ducts
   c. Tenderness
   d. Pain
4. Is the mother holding the infant correctly?
   a. Supports head and body
   b. Brings infant close
   c. Supports breast with other hand using C hold
5. Is infant sucking correctly?
   a. Lips tightly around the full areola
   b. Jaws moving up and down in a rhythmic pattern
6. Is infant's tongue under nipple?
7. Assess infant's level of activity.
   a. Sleepy
   b. Crying
   c. Sucking on fists

FOCUS ASSESSMENT—MOTHER

Determine knowledge level regarding breast-feeding.

Determine maternal desire or motivation for breast-feeding.

Observe mother's facial expression and body language during breast-feeding. Monitor mother's state of comfort.

Note position assumed for breast-feeding.

Examine mother's positioning of infant for feeding.

Note infant response to appropriate stimulation, e.g., rooting reflex, sucking pattern and effectiveness.

Examine placement of nipple in infant's mouth.

Monitor indicators of infant intake, e.g., voiding, weight gain, sleep patterns, behaviors while awake.

COMMON PROBLEMS WITH BREAST-FEEDING*

Problem	Prevention	Treatment
PAINFUL NIPPLES	Make sure most of areola is in infant's mouth so he or she does not chew on the nipple.	If fissures, erosions, or blisters develop, assess mother for proper nipple care.
	Change nursing positions with each feeding so that different areas of the nipple are subjected to the greatest stress from sucking.	Expose nipple to a lamp with 40-watt bulb for 15 to 20 minutes. Ice can be applied to painful nipples just before feeding. Ice may interfere with letdown in some mothers.
	Do not allow breasts to become engorged so that the infant has difficulty grasping the nipple. Feed the infant on demand so he or she does not become overly hungry, causing him or her to suck the nipple too vigorously. Start each feeding on alternate breasts so that both breasts are subjected to vigorous sucking that occurs at beginning of feeding.	If symptoms of breast abscess or mastitis develop, i.e., warmth, tenderness, redness, fever, consult primary care provider for probable antibiotic treatment. If painful nipples burn and itch, assess infant for thrush. Consult primary care provider for medication for mother and infant.

ENGORGEMENT	Signs and symptoms of engorgement: taut, shiny reddened breasts; pain, which may extend to axillae (usually disappears in 24-48 hr); no fever.
Encourage infant to suck frequently. Encourage letdown reflex (relaxation, warm drinks, warm shower).	If engorgement occurs, massage breasts toward the nipple before feedings to soften breasts and make grasping nipples easier for infant. Applying hot packs or taking hot shower improves flow of milk. Massage different areas of breast without removing infant from breast, especially in areas where lumps are noted.
Empty alveoli of milk at each feeding. Allow infant to nurse in response to filling of mother's breasts as well as when infant is hungry.	
Express small amounts of milk to soften the areola enough for infant to grasp nipple.	Wear well-fitting supportive bra. The primary care provider may order aspirin, acetaminophen, or codeine for pain relief.

---

* Nursing goal is to teach mother about these potential problems and self-care before discharge.

INTERVENTION

CLIENT SELF-CARE EDUCATION: POSITIONING THE INFANT AT THE BREAST

Action

1. Assume a comfortable position.
2. Turn the infant's body toward you.
3. Keep the infant's shoulder and hip in alignment.

4. Support your breast with your hand, with all four fingers below and thumb above. Place all fingers behind the areola.
5. Touch the infant's lower lip with your breast until his or her mouth is wide open.

6. Bring the infant close to your body and your breast (bring the infant to the breast, not the breast to the infant).
7. If breast tissue presses against the infant's nose, lift breast slightly or lift the infant's head and legs slightly so they are more horizontal rather than at a downward angle. This allows more space around the nose.

Rationale

1. Facilitates letdown reflex.
2. Infant should not have to turn head to grasp nipple.
3. Even distribution of infant's weight prevents pull on the breast.

4. Helps the infant grasp the nipple.

5. Stimulates the infant to open his or her mouth. Stroking both cheeks of infant is avoided because to do so stimulates rooting reflex on both sides and confuses the infant.

6. Allows directing the nipple into center of infant's mouth.

7. Breast tissue pressing against the nose causes infant to stop sucking. Changing position of the infant removes breast tissue from against the nose.

CLIENT SELF-CARE EDUCATION: EXPRESSION OF BREAST MILK

Action

1. Wash hands with warm water and soap.

Rationale

1. Removes pathogens and prevents contamination of nipples with pathogens from hands.

CLIENT SELF-CARE EDUCATION: EXPRESSION OF BREAST MILK—continued

Action	Rationale
2. Prepare equipment; obtain (from nursery) a sterile wide-mouthed container and sterile bottle and cap if milk is to be fed to the infant.	2. Prevents contamination of breast milk with microorganisms.
3. Take a warm shower, have a warm drink, or massage the breasts.	3. Stimulates letdown and flow of milk.
4. Use one hand to support the breast and express the milk; usually the right hand is used for the left breast and left hand for right breast. The other hand is used to hold the container.	4. Helps mother discover the most comfortable position to use.
5. Place forefinger below and thumb above the outer edge of the areola.	5. Places fingers on lactiferous sinuses.
6. Using gentle but firm pressure toward the chest wall, move finger and thumb toward each other; then draw fingers forward with a milking motion.	6. Forces out milk in a stream as the finger and thumb are brought together and released, compressing the area of the lactiferous sinuses between them.
7. Reposition thumb and forefinger, moving in a clockwise direction; then repeat expression of milk.	7. Removes milk from all sinuses.
8. Avoid pulling, pinching, or squeezing motions.	8. Prevents potential damage or bruises to breast tissue.
9. If milk is to be fed to infant, pour into sterile nursing bottle and label with infant's name, the time, and the date. Refrigerate immediately.	9. Breast milk may be refrigerated for up to 48 hours or frozen up to 2 weeks. If a refrigerator is not available, the breast milk can be retained and transported in ice in a small picnic type cooler brought with the mother for this purpose.

CLIENT SELF-CARE EDUCATION: FEEDING FORMULA TO AN INFANT

Action	Rationale
1. Assume a comfortable position sitting up in bed or in a comfortable chair with adequate arm support.	1. A comfortable position helps mother relax and enjoy the feeding.
2. Hold infant close to body in a semireclining position. Tilt bottle enough that milk fills the nipple.	2. Air that is swallowed can rise to top of infant's stomach and be expelled.
3. If the infant does not open mouth readily, gently stroke the lips with nipple.	3. Stroking the lips elicits the rooting reflex and stimulates the infant to open his or her mouth.
4. Place nipple well into mouth on top of the tongue.	4. Some infants elevate their tongue when opening their mouths.
5. As infant sucks, note if air bubbles rise in the bottle.	5. Indicates infant is getting milk. If there are no air bubbles, check to see if nipple is clogged.
6. Bubble infant after he or she takes approximately ½ ounce of formula. Bubble by holding infant upright on your shoulder or holding infant in a sitting position while stroking or patting his or her back.	6. Regurgitation is common during first days of feeding. Some causes are mucus in the stomach, feeding too rapidly, or overfeeding. Vomiting more than two feedings in a row or projectile vomiting is reported to the primary health care provider. Placing infant in a sitting position during bubbling allows better observation of him or her.
7. Feed for 15 to 20 min.	7. A longer feeding may tire the infant; a shorter feeding may not satisfy his or her sucking needs.

CLIENT SELF-CARE EDUCATION: PREPARATION OF FORMULA

Action

1. Wash hands well before starting.

2. If canned formula is used, wash the top of the can with soap and water, using friction, and then thoroughly rinse with hot water.

3. Wash all equipment thoroughly in warm soapy water. A bottle and nipple brush should be used and water squeezed through the nipple to make sure no milk particles or residue remain. Equipment is thoroughly rinsed to remove all traces of soap or detergent.

4. Cover opened cans of formula or milk with foil or plastic wrap and store in the refrigerator. Opened formula must be used within 48 hr.

Rationale

1. Removes pathogens from hands.

2. Removes dust and pathogens from can.

3. Milk particles occlude nipple openings. Using clean dry equipment reduces possibility of growth of bacteria.

4. Covering opened formula protects it from pathogens transmitted through dust or air. Growth of bacteria is likely after milk is open for 48 hr.

Nursing Care Plan

Infant and Mother Who Are Breast-Feeding

Ineffective Breast-Feeding—Related to Lack of Prior Experience and Information

Goals (expected outcomes)	Interventions	Rationale	Evaluation
Mother and infant will demonstrate successful breast-feeding behaviors.	Assist mother with breast-feeding.	Allows nurse to identify and correct errors in breast-feeding techniques.	Mother identifies "hungry" behaviors accurately.
	Discuss feeding behaviors of the term newborn.	Enables mother to identify signs of hunger and respond appropriately to meet infant's needs.	Infant "latches on" correctly, sucks vigorously. Baby empties breasts every 2 to 3 hours.
	Put newborn to breast when he/she demonstrates "hungry" behaviors (e.g., sucking fist).	Increases potential for successful breast-feeding.	Mother expresses satisfaction with breast-feeding.
	Help mother to position self comfortably.	Comfortable position facilitates relaxation; maternal tension or pain inhibits the let-down reflex.	
	Moisten nipple with a small amount of expressed colostrum or milk.	Scent of colostrum stimulates infant rooting.	

	Help mother to position the infant with his/her body turned toward her breast and his/her mouth covering the areola.	Facilitates "latching-on". Allows effective sucking to compress the ducts and eject milk.

ALTERED NUTRITION: LESS THAN BODY REQUIREMENTS—RELATED TO INFANT'S INEFFECTIVE SUCKING TECHNIQUE

Infant will nurse for at least 10 min every 2 to 3 hrs.	Assist mother with breast-feeding.	Allows nurse to identify and correct errors in breast-feeding techniques.	Infant "latches-on" easily and correctly; sucks vigorously.
	Verify placement of mother's nipple in infant's mouth.	Facilitates "latching-on" and effective sucking to empty breasts into the infant's mouth.	Infant nurses for at least 10 minutes every 2 to 3 hr.
	Encourage frequent (every 2 to 3 hrs) feedings.	Feeding offered at times when infant usually is hungry.	Infant wets 4 to 6 diapers daily. Sleeps well. Weight loss does not exceed 5% to 10% of birth weight. Regains birth weight within 7 to 10 days after birth.
	Describe signs that infant is receiving adequate nutrition, i.e., voiding, sleeping, weight gain.	Voiding reflects state of hydration. Undisturbed sleep intervals indicate hunger has been satisfied. Weight gain demonstrates nutritional needs are being met.	

MATERNAL
COMPLICATIONS

Chapter 13

HIGH-RISK PREGNANCY

A high-risk pregnancy is one in which the mother or her baby has increased chance of death or disability occurring before, during, or after birth. The nurse, midwife, or physician is responsible for making a careful assessment and evaluating every pregnant woman who presents herself for care.

INDICATORS OF PRENATAL RISK

Risk score	Risk indicator
	DEMOGRAPHIC FACTORS
2	Maternal Age: 15 or under, 35 or over
1	Parity: Nulliparous
2	Grand multipara
1	Race: Nonwhite
1	Marital status: Out of wedlock
1	Economic status: Dependent on public assistance
2	Prenatal care: First visit after 27 weeks or less than five visits
	OBSTETRIC FACTORS
1	Infertility factors: <2 yr
2	>2 yr
1	Previous abortion: One
2	Two or more
	Premature or low birth weight infant:
1	History of one
5	History of two or more
7	This pregnancy

Risk factors have been assigned a weighted number from 7 (highest) to 1 (lowest). A total score of 7 or more places the woman in the high-risk category. Patients identified as high risk should be referred for consultation or intensified prenatal care.

From Edwards L et al: Simplified antepartum risk-scoring system. Obstet Gynecol 5(2):238, 1979.

Reprinted with permission from The American College of Obstetricians and Gynecologists.

INDICATORS OF PRENATAL RISK—continued

**Risk
score** **Risk indicator**

OBSTETRIC FACTORS—cont'd

Previous excessive size infant:
1   One
2   Two or more
5   Previous perinatal loss: One
7   Two or more
7   Postterm, beyond 42 weeks: This pregnancy
5   Previous cesarean delivery
1   Previous congenital anomaly
7   Incompetent cervix
5   Uterine anomaly
2   Contracted pelvis
1   Abnormal presentation: History of
7   This pregnancy
7   Rh negative, sensitized
7   Polyhydramnios
1   Preeclampsia, mild: History of
3   This pregnancy
2   Preeclampsia, severe: History of
7   This pregnancy
1   Multiple pregnancy: History of
7   This pregnancy

MISCELLANEOUS FACTORS

1   Nutrition: More than 20% overweight
5   Massive obesity
2   More than 10% under-weight
3   Poor nutrition
5   Inadequate weight gain (<12 pounds)
3   Excessive weight gain (>48 pounds)
1   Smoking more than one pack/day
1   Drug or alcohol abuse: History of
                            This pregnancy

MEDICAL FACTORS

1   Anemia: 8-10 g
2   <8 g
2   Sickle cell trait
7   Sickle cell disease

Continued

INDICATORS OF PRENATAL RISK—continued

**Risk
score** **Risk indicator**

MEDICAL FACTORS—cont'd

Risk score	Risk indicator
2	Hypertension: Mild
7	Severe
2	Heart disease: Class I or II
5	Class III or IV
7	Heart failure: History of
7	This pregnancy
3	Diabetes: Gestational
7	Overt
1	Thyroid disease: History of
7	This pregnancy
	Venereal disease
1	Gonorrhea or syphilis: History of
5	This pregnancy
3	Cervical neoplasia
	Urinary tract infection
1	afebrile: History of
3	This pregnancy
	Urinary tract infection
2	Febrile: History of
5	This pregnancy
	Psychiatric or neurologic problem:
1	History of
1	This pregnancy
	Other medical condition (e.g., pulmonary disease, severe influenza):
1	History of
5	This pregnancy

RISK SCORE

_____   At first visit
_____   At 36 weeks
_____   On admission to labor and delivery

FACTORS INDICATING THE ADOLESCENT POSSIBLY AT RISK FOR COMPLICATIONS*

Age 16 years or less
Anemia
Poor physical state (e.g., obesity, low weight for height)
Any sexually transmitted disease
Use of tobacco, alcohol, or street drugs
Poverty
Lack of social support
Prior medical conditions that pregnancy may complicate (e.g., diabetes, epilepsy, asthma)

FOCUS ASSESSMENT—PREGNANT ADOLESCENT

Identify current knowledge level regarding:
    Potential impact of pregnancy on present and future plans
    Options and access to available resources
    Common pregnancy-related changes
    Anticipated needs and desired pregnancy-related behaviors
Determine current coping behaviors.
Identify current life-style and problem-solving abilities.
Determine adequacy of support system.
Monitor frequency of and interval between prenatal visits.
Monitor pregnancy progress closely (e.g., vital signs, weight gain, fundal height).

---

*From Foster RR, Hunsberger MM, Anderson JJT: Family Centered Nursing Care of Children. Philadelphia, WB Saunders, 1989.

ASSESSMENT OF FETAL STATUS

SUMMARY OF HIGH-RISK SCREENING AND DIAGNOSTIC TESTS

Test purpose	Test used	When test may be done
To determine amounts of amniotic fluid present	Ultrasound for gestational sac volume	5 and 6 wk after last menstrual period
To determine how advanced the pregnancy is	Ultrasound: Crown-rump length Ultrasound: Biparietal diameter and femur length	7-10 wk gestation 13-40 wk gestation
To identify normal growth of the fetus	Ultrasound: Biparietal diameter	Most useful 20-30 wk gestation
	Ultrasound: Head-abdomen ratio Ultrasound: Estimated fetal weight	13-40 wk gestation Approximately 28-40 wk gestation
To detect congenital anomalies and problems	Ultrasound Chorionic villus sampling Fetoscopy Percutaneous blood sampling	18-40 wk gestation 8-12 wk gestation 18 wk gestation Second and third trimesters
To locate the placenta	Ultrasound	Usually in third trimester or before amniocentesis

To assess fetal status	Biophysical profile	Approximately 28 wk to delivery
	Maternal assessment of fetal activity	Approximately 27 wk to delivery
	Estriol determination	During second and third trimesters
	Magnetic resonance imaging	During second and third trimesters
	Nonstress test	Approximately 30 wk to delivery
	Contraction stress test	Last few wk of gestation
To diagnose cardiac problems	Fetal echocardiography	Second and third trimesters
To assess fetal lung maturity	Amniocentesis	33 to 40 wk
	LS ratio	33 wk to delivery
	Phosphatidylglycerol	33 wk to delivery
	Phosphatidylcholine	33 wk to delivery
	Shake test	33 wk to delivery
To obtain more information about breech presentation	Computerized tomography and radiography	Just before labor is anticipated or during labor

SOME INDICATIONS FOR USING ULTRASOUND IN ASSESSMENT OF THE HIGH-RISK FETUS

Estimation of gestational age

Evaluation of fetal growth and development

Evaluation of suspected multiple gestation

Diagnosis of ectopic pregnancy, pelvic mass, or hydatidiform mole

Determination of location of placenta

Evaluation of fetal condition, especially if suspected fetal death

Identification of fetal anomalies

Aid to proper placement of needle in amniocentesis

Aid to special procedures such as fetoscopy or intrauterine transfusion

NURSING PROCEDURE: ULTRASOUND

Intervention	**Rationale**
1. Explain the procedure to the client.	Ultrasound is a painless procedure that uses sound waves to visualize the baby and placenta. No radiation (or x-ray) is used that could harm the baby. Much information is provided to the doctor about the size, age, growth, and well-being of the baby and the placement and maturity of the placenta.
2. Instruct the woman to drink at least 1 quart of water (4-5 cups) approximately 2 hr before the test if a transabdominal ultrasound is to be performed.	When the bladder is full, other pelvic structures can be identified in relation to the bladder. If a vaginal probe is used, the bladder is emptied.
3. Instruct the woman not to empty her bladder before the test.	The woman may feel discomfort because of the full bladder, so care must be taken so she is not kept waiting.

NURSING PROCEDURE: ULTRASOUND—continued

Intervention

4. If the bladder is not sufficiently filled, she is asked to drink another quart of fluid and is rescanned again 30 to 45 min later.
5. Gel is spread on the abdomen.
6. The sonographer moves a transducer across the abdomen for 20-30 min to obtain a picture of the uterine contents.
7. The woman lies on her back during the test.

8. Allow the client and her significant other to view the screen during the procedure.
9. Give verbal explanation and reassurance during the test.
10. Cleanse gel from the abdomen after the procedure.

Rationale

Gel aids transmission of the sound waves.

If the woman experiences shortness of breath, her upper body may be elevated.

Gel is sticky and may adhere to the clothing.

NURSING PROCEDURE: AMNIOCENTESIS WITH ULTRASOUND

Intervention	Rationale
1. Confirm informed consent.	1. Demonstrates ethical, legal accountability to client, physician, hospital, staff

2. Explain procedure step by step.
   a. Ultrasound
   b. Amniocentesis
   c. Post procedure care
	2. Reduces anxiety; enables cooperation

3. Encourage client to drink three to four glasses of water or other fluids 1 hr before procedure. Instruct client not to void. Inform her she may experience some discomfort from a full bladder.	3. Fills bladder to enhance transmission of sound waves and visualization of uterus
4. Assemble all equipment; prepare labels for specimen containers.	4. Facilitates effective, efficient completion of procedure
5. Immediately before procedure, take blood pressure and fetal heart rate.	5. Provides baseline for comparison

6. Place client in supine position.
   a. Instruct client to fold her hands on her chest or place them over her head.
   b. Remind client to remain still throughout the procedure.
   c. If procedure is performed in later pregnancy, may elevate right hip on small pillow.
	6. Facilitates locating placenta and fetus with Doppler
	   a. Reduces risk of accidental contamination by client
	   b. Reduces risk of injury to client or fetus
	   c. Minimizes the potential for supine hypotensive (vena caval) syndrome

7. Ultrasonographer will coat abdomen with conductive gel.	7. Enables transmission of sound waves

Nursing Action	Rationale
8. Transducer is passed vertically and horizontally across the client's abdomen.	8. Locates position of fetus, placenta, and pocket(s) of amniotic fluid; verifies fetal life; minimizes risk of injury to fetus, placenta, or maternal organs
9. If assisting with the procedure, mask, scrub, gown, and glove while ultrasound is in progress.	9. This is a sterile procedure
10. Cleanse abdomen with antiseptic solution.	10. Removes surface microorganisms; reduces risk of infection
11. Drape client's abdomen.	11. Maintains sterile field
12. Assist as directed, maintaining sterile technique.	12. Facilitates effective, efficient completion of sterile procedure
a. If requested, prepare sterile syringe with local anesthetic.	a. Physician may use local anesthetic to reduce client discomfort from needle insertion
b. Provide sterile 20- or 22-gauge spinal needle with stylette in place. Ready sterile 20 to 30 cc syringe for use.	b. Size appropriate to aspirate fluid with minimum tissue trauma
c. Open sterile specimen tubes; prepare to receive specimen.	c. Contamination can cause chromosomal aberrations
d. Physician will discard first 5 ml of fluid.	d. May contain maternal cells
e. Collect sterile specimen; cap tubes tightly.	e. Protects specimen from contamination or spilling
13. When physician withdraws needle, remove drapes and apply adhesive bandage over insertion site.	13. Protects puncture wound
14. Complete laboratory request slips; send specimen to laboratory immediately.	14. Assures prompt, appropriate treatment of specimen

Continued

NURSING PROCEDURE: AMNIOCENTESIS WITH ULTRASOUND—continued

Intervention	Rationale
15. Monitor maternal vital signs and fetal heart rate every 15 min for 30 min or for 1 to 2 hr (according to hospital protocol).	15. Detects changes from baseline; identifies early signs of complications; ensures prompt treatment
16. Instruct client to notify physician promptly of a. Vaginal discharge of fluid or blood b. Decreased fetal movement c. Contractions d. Fever, chills	16. Assures prompt evaluation of maternal and fetal status
17. Complete client record.	17. Documents procedure instructions given and client status at discharge

Sample narrative charting: Postamniocentesis. Alert and responsive. No complaint of pain. Bandage applied to site. Bandage dry and intact. Resting on examining table. Temperature 98.8°F (oral), BP 110/76, P 68, R 16. FHR LLQ 136. Instructions reviewed regarding reporting of bleeding, fever, or leakage of amniotic fluid. Verbalized understanding of how to contact Dr. Edmiston.

NONSTRESS TEST

Purpose
Demonstrates that FHR increases normally with movement.

Results
Reactive: FHR accelerations are present, indicating a healthy fetus.
Nonreactive: Normal accelerations are not present with movement, or lack of fetal movement may mean the fetus is sleeping or compromised. Further evaluation is indicated.

CONTRACTION STRESS TEST

Purpose
Evaluates the reaction of the FHR to induced or spontaneous contractions.

Results
Negative (desired test outcome): No late deceleration of the FHR when an adequate frequency of three contractions in 10 min has been established.
Positive: Occurrence of late decelerations with three contractions in 10 min.
Unsatisfactory test: Inadequate contractions or FHR records.

EFFECTS OF DIABETES MELLITUS ON PREGNANCY

Effects on mother	Effects on fetus or neonate
Fourfold increase of pregnancy-induced hypertension	High perinatal mortality rate
Infection, commonly severe	Birth trauma caused by large size
Dystocia caused by large baby	Fourfold increase of congenital, especially cardiac, anomalies
Hydramnios	Postnatal hypoglycemia
Increased frequency of cesarean section	Polycythemia
Postpartum hemorrhage	Hyperbilirubinemia

Blood Tests Used in Diagnosing Diabetes

Fasting blood sugar (FBS): Test used to determine the amount of glucose remaining in the blood after a period of fasting. Two elevations >140 mg/dl are indicative of diabetes mellitus.

Two hour postprandial test: A more sensitive test but not considered totally diagnostic of diabetes.

Oral glucose tolerance test (OGTT): Considered positive if plasma glucose concentration is 200 mg/dl or higher 1 to 2 hr after a measured intake of oral glucose.

Intravenous glucose tolerance test (IGTT): Preferred test in pregnancy because glucose absorption from the intestinal tract may vary and alter findings of OGTT.

Principles of Management of Diabetes During Pregnancy*

Principle 1: Strict control of maternal glucose levels

Principle 2: Prompt detection and treatment of maternal complications

Principle 3: Fetal surveillance, including diagnosis of fetal macrosomia

Principle 4: Avoidance of unnecessary premature delivery

Assessment

Diabetes in Pregnancy

Ask client while obtaining nursing history if she has any of the risk factors for diabetes:

Previous infant weighing more than 9 pounds

Previous pregnancy loss

Previous neonatal death, stillbirth, anomaly, or premature infant

Family history of diabetes mellitus or previous gestational diabetes

History of hypertension or recurrent urinary tract infections or candidiasis

---

*Modified from Gibbons JM: Diabetes in pregnancy. In Schnatz JD (ed): Diabetes Mellitus: Problems in Management. Menlo Park, Calif, Addison-Wesley, 1982.

At each prenatal visit observe client for the following:

Weight gain

Glucosuria on two or more visits

Fundal height greater than expected for gestation

Signs of diabetes

Polyuria beyond first trimester and before third trimester

Polydipsia

Polyphagia

Weight loss

If diabetes is diagnosed, assess client's knowledge of the following:

Signs and symptoms of hypoglycemia

Signs and symptoms of hyperglycemia

Signs and symptoms of urinary tract infections or candidiasis

Self-care, including diet and insulin if needed

FOCUS ASSESSMENT—PREGNANT DIABETIC

Identify when client first developed symptoms.

Determine specific learning needs, e.g., prenatal diabetic diet, capillary blood glucose testing (CBG), signs and symptoms of hyperglycemia and hypoglycemia.

Monitor blood glucose levels (patient report, lab report, CBGs)

Explore complaints that suggest complications of pregnancy, e.g., hyperemesis, threatened abortion, premature labor, or infection.

As pregnancy progresses:

Monitor fundal height for indications of fetal macrosomia, hydramnios.

Monitor fetal status, e.g., nonstress testing.

ASSESSMENT

HEART DISEASE IN PREGNANCY

1. Ask client to describe the following:
   a. Ability to perform various types of physical activities before pregnancy
   b. Dyspnea on exertion
   c. Coughing
   d. Palpitations
2. At each prenatal visit assess the following:
   a. Heart and breath sounds
   b. Edema and tenderness of extremities
   c. Baseline vital signs and FHR
   d. Symptoms of cardiac decompression: coughing and hemoptysis, dyspnea or orthopnea, edema, heart murmurs, palpitations, rales
3. Note results of tests and report to physician:
   a. Chest x-ray examination
   b. Electrocardiogram

FOCUS ASSESSMENT—PREGNANT CLIENT WITH HEART DISEASE

Determine current cardiac status and management.

Identify number of weeks gestation.

Monitor vital signs closely.

Explore complaints of fatigue with usual activities, dyspnea, sleep pattern disturbance, signs of infection.

CONGENTIAL DISORDERS CAUSED BY MATERNAL TORCH DISEASES

Disease	Transmission	Mother	Fetus or infant	Medical intervention	Nursing interventions
Toxoplasmosis caused by a protozoa, *Toxoplasma gondii*	Placental transfer Handling cat litter contaminated with feces containing oocytes (from unconfined cats) Eating poorly cooked or raw meat	Generally asymptomatic Primary infection acquired just before or during early pregnancy May result in congenital infection May result in spontaneous abortion	Death in 10% to 15% Classic congenital defects: chorioretinitis, microcephaly, hydrocephalus, cerebral calcifications	IgG and IgM antibody testing in cord and neonatal blood; drugs of choice: pyrimethamine, sulfadiazine	Counsel pregnant woman to avoid emptying cat litter from unconfined cats and to avoid ingestion of partially cooked or raw meat. Special isolation precautions are not needed.
Rubella caused by a virus	Across the placenta Fetus vulnerable during first trimester and early second trimester if mother contracts rubella	Spontaneous abortion in 33% of pregnant women with rubella in first trimester	Cardiac defects, cataracts, deafness	Testing for rubella-specific IgM from cord or neonatal serum; immediate serologic testing for exposed women	Affected babies and their placentas are highly infected. Nonimmune personnel, especially pregnant women, should avoid con-

Continued

CONGENITAL DISORDERS CAUSED BY MATERNAL TORCH DISEASES—continued

Disease	Transmission	Mother	Fetus or infant	Medical intervention	Nursing interventions
				Perinatal rubella rare in United States because of immunization programs; nonimmune women followed carefully for clinical rubella or development of antibodies. Immunization and gamma globulin not recommended	tact. Immunity status of all personnel is determined and vaccination administered at the time of employment. Provide strict isolation for affected infants. Infants may be isolated with their mothers in a private room.
Infection caused by cytomegalovirus (CMV)—	Across the placenta. Contaminated vaginal or nasopharyngeal se-	Asymptomatic	Many asymptomatic Bone lesions, low birth weight, ane-	Diagnostic studies: viral cultures of amniotic fluid or neonatal serum; anti-CMV IgM	Counsel pregnant women to avoid close contact with known cases.

most common of perinatal viruses	cretions, urine, or feces. Less frequently, blood transfusions or breast milk	mia, jaundice, hepatosplenomegaly	antibodies in cord or neonatal serum; CMV inclusion in urine or cerebrospinal fluid. Treatment is supportive	Counsel parents that CMV may be found in affected infant's urine for a number of years. Teach parents appropriate disposal of diapers and handwashing after diapering.
Hepatitis B caused by specific hepatitis B virus	Infection of infants during last trimester or during delivery. During postpartum period through infected maternal saliva, urine, feces, serum, breast milk	Malaise, fever, jaundice, dark urine, light stools, anorexia. Low birth weight if affected in utero. May be asymptomatic if infected at time of delivery	Diagnostic studies: hepatitis B virus cultured from amniotic fluid; IgM in cord blood or neonatal serum. Administration of hepatitis B immunoglobin to infants of infected mothers	Follow enteric, blood, and secretion precautions.

Continued

CONGENITAL DISORDERS CAUSED BY MATERNAL TORCH DISEASES—continued

Disease	Transmission	Mother	Fetus or infant	Medical intervention	Nursing interventions
Fifth disease (erythema infectiosum, slap-cheek disease) caused by human *Parvovirus 19*	Through air from person to person Infectious period uncertain, probably only in prodromal period	Rash, fever, chills, joint pain	Increased incidence of stillbirth and abortion in women with this disease during pregnancy	Detected by specific antigen-antibody testing No vaccine available Identification of recent infections through IgM tests No specific treatment	Counsel pregnant women to avoid persons with febrile diseases, especially if known outbreak. Counsel pregnant women to report febrile diseases with rashes.

Chapter 14

ANTEPARTUM COMPLICATIONS

Pregnancy-related maternal disorders are divided into two broad categories: (1) complications related to the pregnancy itself and not seen at other times and (2) diseases that are not pregnancy-related but occur coincidentally. The latter may arise in the non-pregnant woman as well, but when they occur during pregnancy, they may complicate the pregnancy and influence its course or may be aggravated by the pregnancy.

COMPLICATIONS EARLY IN PREGNANCY

Complications occurring early in pregnancy include: abortion, incompetent cervix, ectopic pregnancy, hyperemesis, gravidarium, and hydatidiform mole.

TYPES OF ABORTION

Spontaneous: Process occurs through natural causes.

Therapeutic: Artificially induced for medical or other reasons.

Threatened: Bleeding and/or cramping occurs, but cervix is closed. Pregnancy may or may not be lost.

Inevitable: Bleeding and cramping with dilating cervix.

Incomplete: Part of products of conception are passed, but part are retained. Bleeding usually persists until uterus is empty.

Complete: Expulsion of all products of conception.

Missed: Fetus dies in utero but is retained.

Habitual: Three or more pregnancies are lost in succession.

Illegal: Termination of pregnancy outside of appropriate medical facilities, generally by nonphysician abortionists. Each state has statutes that define the parameters that constitute an illegal abortion in that particular state.

ASSESSMENT

BLEEDING IN EARLY PREGNANCY: INITIAL DATA BASE

The initial data base should be completed at time of admission to the hospital.

Chief complaint: Why are you here?

Vital signs:

Gravida and parity:

Date of last menstrual period:

Estimated date of confinement:

Pregnancy history (previous abortion, ectopic, etc.):

Allergies:

Current pregnancy confirmed:

Nausea and vomiting:

Type of pain: contractions, cramping backache, abdominal pain (dull or sharp)

Onset of pain:

Previous bleeding or coagulation problems:

Quantity of bleeding: (e.g., teaspoon, ½ cup)

Nature of blood loss: bright red to dark brown (with or without tissue fragments)

When bleeding began: intermittent or continuous

Dizziness:

Patient anxiety:

Emotional status: What does the loss mean to you?

Sample Narrative Charting: Admitted per stretcher complaining of severe cramping and excessive bleeding since early this morning. Has saturated 9 maxi pads (¾ of pad each time) in past 6 hours and has passed several 50-cent piece size clots. No tissue seen. Presently there is a large amount of bright red bleeding (2 pads thoroughly soaked in 20 minutes). Cramping is intermittent at 3- to 4-minute intervals. Feels some rectal pressure. Nothing seen at introitus. Temperature 97.6° F. Blood pressure 80/40, pulse 120 and thready, respirations 24 and shallow. Skin is clammy and perspiring. States "Every time I lift my head I feel very dizzy." Dr. Edmiston called and given report.

FOCUS ASSESSMENT—SPONTANEOUS ABORTION

Estimate number of weeks gestation.

Monitor vital signs closely.

Monitor vaginal bleeding:

    Maintain perineal pad count.

    Note degree of saturation.

    Identify signs of increasing or decreasing bleeding.

Examine any clots or tissue discharged.

Elicit description of pain (type, persistence); note any changes.
Elicit information describing perception of self.
Explore nonverbal indicators of emotional status, e.g., irritability, inability to concentrate, withdrawal.

ASSESSMENT

FOCUS ASSESSMENT—INCOMPETENT CERVIX

Elicit information describing perception of self.
Explore nonverbal indicators of emotional status, e.g., affect, mood, inability to concentrate.
Identify previous patterns of coping with crisis.
Determine current support system.

ASSESSMENT

FOCUS ASSESSMENT—ECTOPIC PREGNANCY

Monitor vital signs closely.
Identify nonverbal signs of pain, anxiety, fear.
Elicit description of pain (type, persistence); note any changes.
Examine intake and output balance.
Indentify individual teaching or learning needs.
Monitor response to analgesia and anesthesia.
Elicit information describing perception of self.
Explore nonverbal indicators of emotional status, e.g., irritability, inability to concentrate, withdrawal.

ASSESSMENT

BLEEDING IN LATE PREGNANCY

Gravida, para, abortion:
Estimated date of confinement:
LMP:
Quantity of bleeding: (e.g., teaspoon, ½ cup)
What precipitated bleeding:
Pain associated with bleeding: (uterine contractions, backache)
Amniotic sac: (ruptured, intact)
Uterine activity and condition: (size, contour, irritability, relaxation)
Abdominal pain: (dull, sharp, knifelike)

Vital signs:

Fetal activity:

Fetal heart rate:

General status: (level of consciousness, dizzy, apprehensive, anxious)

FOCUS ASSESSMENT—BLEEDING IN LATE PREGNANCY

Monitor vital signs and fetal heart rate closely.

Estimate amount of blood loss. Identify signs of increase or decrease in bleeding.

Monitor level of consciousness.

Identify presence or absence of pain.

When pain is present, note changes in character, amount, site, and response to pain.

Explore nonverbal indicators of emotional status, e.g., affect, mood, appearance, irritability, inability to concentrate, sleep patterns.

Identify expectations of pregnancy outcome.

Determine individual teaching or learning needs.

Observe family interactions.

COMPARATIVE OVERVIEW OF PLACENTA PREVIA AND ABRUPTIO PLACENTAE

	Placenta previa	Abruptio placentae
Etiology	Unknown	Unknown
Associated risk factors	Multiparity, multiple gestation, advancing age (over 35), uterine incisions, previous cesarean section	Multiparity, chronic hypertension, PIH, uterine trauma, short umbilical cord, uterine anomaly, (perhaps) folic acid deficiency
Frequency	1 : 167 deliveries	1 : 77 to 1 : 200 deliveries
Symptoms	Painless bleeding, soft uterus, observable blood loss comparable to that with signs of shock	Sudden, intense, localized uterine pain with or without bleeding Shock out of proportion to observable blood loss

COMPARATIVE OVERVIEW OF PLACENTA PREVIA AND ABRUPTIO PLACENTAE—continued

	Placenta previa	**Abruptio placentae**
Prognosis	Maternal mortality: 0.1% Major problem: prematurity Perinatal mortality: 15%-20%	Maternal mortality: 0.5%-5% Perinatal mortality: 15%
Recurrence	1:17	1:6 to 1:18
Complications	Hemorrhage Hypovolemic shock Thrombocytopenia Premature rupture of membranes Fetal malposition Air embolism Postpartum hemorrhage Uterine rupture	Hemorrhage DIC Renal failure Anemia Pulmonary embolus

CLASSIFICATION OF ABRUPTIO PLACENTAE ACCORDING TO PLACENTAL SEPARATION

Mild

Minimum placental separation (less than one-sixth of placenta is separated)
Bleeding: less than 500 ml
Maternal condition: good
Fetal condition: good
No special intervention

Moderate

Bleeding: 500-1000 ml
Maternal condition: cardiovascular instability
Fetal condition: FHR may or may not be present

Severe

Bleeding: hemorrhage (overt or covert)
Placental separation: more than two-thirds
Maternal condition: unstable (hypotension, tachycardia, DIC, renal failure)
Fetal condition: distress or intrauterine death

CLINICAL STAGING OF HEMORRHAGIC SHOCK BY VOLUME OF BLOOD LOSS

	Mild (20%-25% loss)	Moderate (25-35% loss)	Severe (>35% loss)	Irreversible
Respirations	Rapid, deep	Rapid, becoming shallow	Rapid, shallow, may be irregular	Irregular or barely perceptible
Pulse	Rapid; tone normal	Rapid; tone may be normal but is becoming weaker	Very rapid; easily collapsible; may be irregular	Irregular apical pulse
	<100 bpm	100-120 bpm	>120 bpm	
Blood pressure	Normal or hypertensive	80-100 mm Hg systolic	<60 mm Hg systolic	None palpable
Skin	Cool and pale Peripheral vasoconstriction	Cool, pale, moist; knees cyanotic	Cold, clammy; cyanosis of lips and fingernails	Cold, clammy, cyanotic
Urinary output	No change	Decreasing to 10-22 ml/hr	Oliguric (<10 ml) to anuric	Anuric
Level of consciousness	Alert, oriented; diffuse anxiety	Oriented, mental cloudiness, or increasing restlessness	Lethargy; reacts to noxious stimuli; comatose	Does not respond to noxious stimuli
Central venous pressure	May be normal	3 cm H_2O	0-3 cm H_2O	

bpm—beats per minute.

ASSESSMENT

FOCUS ASSESSMENT—DISSEMINATED INTRAVASCULAR COAGULATION

Monitor vital signs and fetal heart rate closely.

Estimate amount of blood loss. Identify signs of increase or decrease in bleeding.

Monitor level of consciousness.

Identify presence or absence of pain.

Determine individual teaching or learning needs.

Observe family interactions.

Nursing Care Plan

Hemorrhage Occurring in Late Pregnancy

Goals (expected outcomes)	Interventions	Rationale	Evaluation
DECREASED CARDIAC OUTPUT—RELATED TO HYPOVOLEMIA			
The client will maintain adequate cardiac output so perfusion is maintained to brain, kidneys, liver, and uteroplacental unit.	Assess maternal blood loss and vital signs every 15 min to every 1 hr.	Hypotension indicates a large amount of blood loss.	Client's blood loss is controlled, and vital signs are stable.
	Maintain bed rest with client in left-lateral position.	Ensures best blood supply to uterus, placenta, and kidneys.	Client rests comfortably in bed.
	Initiate and monitor intravenous fluids to restore circulating volume (use at least 18-gauge needle).	Restores circulation volume.	Client received adequate fluid intake.
	Type and crossmatch two (or more) units of whole blood.	Replaces blood immediately as needed.	Client returns to normal urinary output.
	Review results of serial CBC, hemoglobin, and hematocrit values.	Indicates amount of blood lost.	Homeostasis is achieved.

Administer oxygen as needed for client and infant.	Increases oxygen saturation.	Both are well-oxygenated; maternal vital signs are normal; and baseline fetal heart rate (FHR) in normal range of 110-160.
Monitor and record intake and output.	Promotes and maintains fluid electrolyte balance.	Fluid and electrolyte balance is maintained.
Count and weigh perineal pads; inspect contents for tissue.	Estimates blood loss. Promotes homeostasis.	Homeostasis is achieved.
Report change in level of consciousness.	May occur with shock.	Client is alert and visiting with mate.
Report presence of pallor, cyanosis, coolness, dampness.	Occurs with shock and loss of hemoglobin.	Color is good; skin is warm and dry with good turgor.
Report change in uterine contractions for frequency, duration, intensity, and resting tone.	Increase may be due to placental separation (no increase with placenta previa).	Contraction pattern is normal, with good relaxation between contractions.
Report change in fundal height.	Concealed bleeding may cause increase in fundal height.	Fundal height is unchanged.

Continued

NURSING CARE PLAN

HEMORRHAGE OCCURRING IN LATE PREGNANCY—continued

Goals (expected outcomes)	Interventions	Rationale	Evaluation
DECREASED CARDIAC OUTPUT—RELATED TO HYPOVOLEMIA—cont'd			
	Monitor CVP for vital functioning.	Monitors adequate return of blood to maternal heart.	Homeostasis is achieved.
	Apply fetal monitor; assess FHR.	Assesses fetus for stress or distress (possibly death).	Fetus has normal baseline FHR (110-160); with good variability and no accelerations and decelerations.
	Prepare for delivery.	Optimizes fetal outcome and controls hemorrhage.	All equipment for initial care and resuscitation is ready and checked.
	Notify neonatologist or pediatrician of impending delivery.	Infant may require care and resuscitation.	Neonatologist or pediatrician is present for delivery.
KNOWLEDGE DEFICIT—REGARDING PHYSIOLOGIC ALTERATIONS IN THE REPRODUCTIVE SYSTEM			
Client will verbalize understanding of performed procedures.	Instruct client about "danger signals" in early pregnancy and what actions to take.	Encourages early recognition and reporting of danger signals.	Client verbalizes danger signals and what to do.

	Instruct client about limiting activity, getting bed rest, and abstaining from sexual activity.	Enables active client participation in own health maintenance.	Client verbalizes why interventions are necessary.
DYSFUNCTIONAL GRIEVING—RELATED TO ACTUAL OR THREATENED LOSS OF PREGNANCY			
Client feels comfortable to grieve as she wishes.	Provide opportunities for expression of grief, anger, loss.	Provides understanding of grieving process.	Client is resolving grief appropriately.
	Allow client to be with supportive family members.	Individuals derive support from family or significant others.	Grief is being shared with supportive individuals.
Client believes support is available in a nonjudgmental atmosphere.	Accept client's feelings of grief and associated behaviors in nonjudgmental manner.	Anger is part of grieving.	Client understands anger in the context of grief.
	Provide factual information about abortion (or ectopic pregnancy or hydatidiform mole) and possible future reproductive capacities.	Fear is greater with unknown.	Client understands information about bleeding.
	Initiate referral for genetic counseling if appropriate.	Information related to recurrence rates is provided.	Client makes arrangements for counseling (genetic) if appropriate.

Continued

NURSING CARE PLAN

HEMORRHAGE OCCURRING IN LATE PREGNANCY—continued

Goals (expected outcomes)	Interventions	Rationale	Evaluation
DYSFUNCTIONAL GRIEVING—RELATED TO ACTUAL OR THREATENED LOSS OF PREGNANCY—cont'd			
	Initiate referral for support services if desired.	Follow-up with support services helps resolve grieving process.	Client is resolving grief process.
INFECTION—RELATED TO RUPTURED MEMBRANES, PROCEDURES			
Client recovers without complications of infection.	Provide education about perineal hygiene.	Proper cleansing helps prevent infection.	Client demonstrates proper cleansing technique after voiding.
	Assess vital signs (especially temperature).	Infection usually causes fever.	Vital signs remain within normal limits.
	Assess for local tenderness.	Sign of postpartum endometrial infection.	Client states has no tenderness or pain.
	Assess for malodorous vaginal discharge.	Sign of infection.	Client has no odor with vaginal discharge.

ASSESSMENT

SICKLE CELL CRISIS

Signs and Symptoms
Joint pain
Laboratory verification of
   RBC sickling
Temperature elevation
Petechiae
Jaundice
Abdominal pain
Hematuria/hemoptysis
Chills

Precipitating Factors
Infection
PIH
Hemolytic and folic acid
   deficiency anemia
Eclampsia
Dehydration

FOCUS ASSESSMENT—SICKLE CELL CRISIS

Determine current level of knowledge regarding her disorder,
   effects of pregnancy on the disorder, effects of the disorder
   on pregnancy, and prenatal management.
Explore nonverbal indicators of affect, mood.
Elicit information regarding self-image.
Monitor hemoglobin and hematocrit values.
Explore complaints that suggest
   Complications of pregnancy, e.g., threatened abortion, preg-
      nancy-induced hypertension, premature labor, or infec-
      tion.
   Complications of sickle cell anemia, e.g., renal dysfunction,
      cardiovascular instability.
Monitor fetal status, e.g., nonstress testing, contraction stress
   testing, ultrasonography.

MANAGEMENT OF UNSENSITIZED Rh-NEGATIVE CLIENT

Initial Visit
Blood group, Rh type, and indirect Coombs' test antibody screen
   are determined.

At 28 Weeks Gestation
Indirect Coombs' test is repeated. If there are no Rh antibodies,
   300 µg of Rh_o (D) immune globulin are administered to provide
   protection for 12 weeks.

At 35 Weeks Gestation

An anti-D (Rh_o) titer is done. If titer is 1 : 4 or greater, it could mean there is active immunization.

At Delivery

The anti-D (Rh_o) titer is repeated. A titer greater than 1 : 4 means the client has active immunization and the client is *not* a candidate for Rh_o (D) immune globulin.

Lower titers indicate client *is* a candidate for Rh_o (D) immune globulin.

Blood grouping, Rh typing, and direct Coombs' test are determined on cord blood.

A Betke-Kleihaner test is ordered if a transplacental bleed is suspected, and its results are used to determine if additional Rh_o (D) immune globulin is required.

HYPERTENSIVE DISORDERS OF PREGNANCY

PREDISPOSING CONDITIONS FOR PIH (PREGNANCY-INDUCED HYPERTENSION)

Before pregnancy	During pregnancy
Diabetes mellitus	Primigravida age extremes (<20 yr or >35 yr)
Hypertension	
Renal disease	Hydramnios
Low income	Multiple gestation
Family history of PIH	Hydatidiform mole
Family history of hypertension or vascular disease	Large fetus
	Glomerulonephritis

LABORATORY DATA RELATED TO PIH

	Normal pregnancy	Pregnancy with PIH
Hemoglobin and hematocrit	12.1-12.7 g/dl 35%-42%	Elevated due to hemo-concentration
Plasma volume	Increased by 45%-50%	Reduced
Uric acid	6 mg/dl	Usually elevated
Serum creatinine	0.6-0.8 mg/dl	Elevated in severe PIH
Blood glucose	70-110 mg/dl	Normal
Electrolytes	Normal	Normal
Glomerular filtration rate	Increases by 50%	Decreased

ASSESSMENT

PIH

Gravida, para, abortions:

Estimated date of confinement:

LMP:

Gestation:

Age:

Marital status:

Prenatal history: (complications of previous pregnancy; complications of present pregnancy)

Previous and present medications and reasons for use:

Prepregnant weight:

Present weight:

Pattern of weight gain:

Fetal activity: (active, decreased fetal movement)

Subjective signs of elevated blood pressure: (frontal headache, blurred vision, seeing spots of flashes of light, muscle twitching, vomiting, epigastric pain)

Vital signs: (blood pressure taken in sitting or left-lateral position)

Edema: (location and amount)

Dipstick results for urinary protein:

Review of laboratory results: (electrolytes, blood urea nitrogen, creatinine, uric acid, aspartate transaminase, magnesium sulfate, CBC, platelets, PT, PTT)

Lung sounds: (rales present, absent)

Central nervous system status: (jittery, muscle twitchings)

Level of consciousness:

Psychologic status: (apprehensive, anxious)

Fetal assessment: (nonstress test for fetal reactivity, contraction stress test for placental-respiratory reserve, amniotic fluid volume [stable, decreased])

FOCUS ASSESSMENT—PIH

Closely monitor: vital signs, weight gain or loss, presence and amount of protein in urine, digital and periorbital edema, fetal heart rate, results of nonstress tests. (Frequency varies with severity of previous assessment findings and change in maternal or fetal status.)

Observe for signs of pathologic progression: deep tendon reflexes, emergence of complaints of headache or epigastric pain, level of consciousness.

Monitor for signs of medication effects: vital signs, deep tendon reflexes, intake and output, weight loss.

Determine current level of knowledge regarding disorder, status, management.

Explore nonverbal indicators of emotional status, e.g., affect, mood, appearance, inability to concentrate, sleep patterns.

Identify expectations of pregnancy outcome.

FETAL ASSESSMENT

For Well-being
Fetal movement (mother records interval of time it takes for 10 fetal movements)
Nonstress testing
Contraction stress testing
Biophysical profile
Ultrasonography for placental grading

For Maturity
Amniocentesis for lecithin/sphingomyelin ratio or phosphotidyl glycerol
Ultrasonographic measurements

SIGNS OF RECOVERY FROM PIH AFTER DELIVERY*

Urinary output of 4-6 L/day for first 2 days
Resolution of edema within 4-5 days
Rapid weight loss
Resolution of proteinurea in approximately 1 wk
Normotensive in approximately 2 wk

---

*If all signs are not absent 4-6 wks after delivery, chronic hypertension is suspected.

INTERVENTION

CLIENT SELF-CARE EDUCATION: PIH: HOME CARE

Intervention

1. Explain necessity of *rest* in left-lateral recumbent position.

2. Explain diet modification: high in protein, avoidance of high-sodium foods, 6-8 glasses of water daily.

3. Instruct client to weigh self daily.

4. Instruct client to report *signs* and *symptoms* of increased severity of PIH.
   a. Decreased urinary output
   b. No weight loss
   c. No decrease or minimum decrease in blood pressure
   d. Headaches, blurred vision, or epigastric pain
   e. Decreasing fetal movement

Rationale

1. This position improves blood flow to kidneys and results in improved glomerular function and placental perfusion.

2. Replaces protein lost in urine and increases urinary output.

3. Determines if amount of edema is changing.

4. Home care is no longer sufficient with increased severity, and hospitalization with more aggressive management is necessary. Depending on gestation, response to medical management, client's well-being or decreasing uteroplacental perfusion, hospitalization may be brief.

CLIENT SELF-CARE EDUCATION: PIH: HOSPITAL CARE

Intervention

1. Explain why hospitalization is necessary.

2. Explain the special diet (70-100 g protein, balanced amount of sodium, and 6-8 glasses of water if urinary output is sufficient).

Rationale

1. Home care is no longer possible if blood pressure continues to rise; proteinuria and edema continue.

2. Special diet will replace protein being lost in urine (must not cheat)

CLIENT SELF-CARE EDUCATION: PIH: HOSPITAL CARE— continued

Intervention	Rationale
3. Explain drugs: a. Phenobarbital	3. a. Barbiturate provides relaxation and rest (in left-lateral position), which are important to facilitate increased blood flow return to client's heart and her cardiac output and uteroplacental perfusion and oxygenation to fetus; also helps mobilize edema.
b. Magnesium sulfate	b. Decreases brain stimulation to reduce possibility of seizures.
c. Hydralazine	c. Decreases blood pressure.
4. Explain why weight is checked daily.	4. Determines whether edema is decreasing or increasing or disease is improving or worsening.
5. Check fluid intake and output daily; give client cups or glasses marked with measures of volume and graduated for measuring output so that she can help in maintaining accurate measurements.	5. Ensures intake and output are appropriate, edema is not increasing, and diuresis is occurring.
6. Explain need for checking blood pressure, pulse, and respiration every 4 hr or as ordered.	6. Determines progress or improvement of PIH.
7. a. Explain need for fetal movement counts and nonstress testing daily.	7. a. Determines fetal well-being
b. Explain need for contraction stress testing by nipple stimulation at least biweekly.	b. Determines respiratory function of placenta and fetal well-being.

CLIENT SELF-CARE EDUCATION: PIH: HOSPITAL CARE—continued

Intervention

8. Explain use of 24-hr urine sample for protein and creatinine determination; explain need to measure and save every voiding.
9. Explain need for drawing blood for laboratory analysis.

10. Explain ultrasound scan.

11. Explain amniocentesis.

12. Explain drug betamethasone.

13. Explain checking of reflexes.
14. Explain ophthalmoscopic examination.

15. If client not too ill, take her by stretcher or wheelchair to newborn intensive care nursery and explain how her infant will be cared for (may explain and use pictures if she is too ill).

Rationale

8. Determines kidney function (helps assess deterioration or improvement of disease process).

9. All laboratory work gives critical information about functioning capacity of maternal kidneys, electrolytes, hemostats, and homeostasis.

10. Determines fetal age and estimates fetal weight.

11. Determines pulmonary lung maturity of fetus.

12. This drug is used to accelerate pulmonary maturity; if fetal lungs are immature but fetus must be delivered, the benefits of delivery outweigh the risks of prematurity.

13. Determines excitability of central nervous system.

14. Shows normal or decreased blood flow to part of brain behind eyes.

15. Helps her know what to expect if infant is born prematurely or requires intensive care and reduces her anxiety and apprehension.

ASSESSMENT

CLINICAL SIGNS AND SYMPTOMS OF IMPENDING ECLAMPSIA

Progression of PIH
Headaches, visual disturbances, epigastric discomfort
Apprehension, excitability
Tachypnea (respiration of 50)
Temperature elevation (103° F)
Increasing proteinuria
Oliguria (less than 30 ml/hr)
Acidosis

FOCUS ASSESSMENT—ECLAMPSIA

Closely monitor vital signs, fetal heart rate, level of consciousness, deep tendon reflexes, intake and output.

Identify signs of impending convulsions: vacant stare, lack of response to verbal stimuli, twitching of facial muscles.

Closely monitor number and severity of convulsions, length of apneic period, depth and duration of coma, return to consciousness.

Identify signs of labor: restlessness at regular intervals during coma, contractions, rupture of membranes, vaginal bleeding.

Explore complaints of abdominal pain.

Closely monitor FHR since convulsions decrease O_2 to fetus already experiencing hypoxia.

NURSING CARE PLAN

CLIENT WITH SEVERE PREGNANCY-INDUCED HYPERTENSION

Goals (expected outcomes)	Interventions	Rationale	Evaluation
POTENTIAL FOR INJURY (MATERNAL)—RELATED TO CNS IRRITABILITY			
Client will respond to treatment without further complications.	Decrease environmental stimuli and limit visitors.	Reduces CNS stimulation.	Client is quiet and relaxed.
	Organize care to minimize disturbing client's rest and quiet.		
	Administer medications as ordered.		
	Phenobarbital	Encourages rest and relaxation.	Client states she rests well.
	Magnesium sulfate	Is a CNS depressant; inhibits convulsions; causes vasodilation and diuresis.	Client exhibits increased urinary output, decreased BP, and normal deep tendon reflexes.
	Apresoline	Causes vasodilation; increases cardiac output and renal flow.	Client exhibits decreased BP.

Continued

Nursing Care Plan

Client with Severe Pregnancy-Induced Hypertension—continued

Goals (expected outcomes)	Interventions	Rationale	Evaluation
POTENTIAL FOR INJURY (MATERNAL)—RELATED TO CNS IRRITABILITY—cont'd			
	Perform client teaching: report any headache, visual disturbances, epigastric pain.	Requires prompt evaluation; may indicate pathologic progression.	Client presents no new signs of progression; all assessment findings are within normal limits.
POTENTIAL FOR INJURY (FETAL)—RELATED TO DIMINISHED UTEROPLACENTAL PERFUSION, HYPOXIA/ANOXIA/ASPHYXIA, PRETERM DELIVERY			
Client experiences a successful gestational outcome.	Encourages woman to rest on left side.	Promotes placental perfusion; protects fetal status.	FHR remains stable between 120 and 160.
	Perform client teaching: Explain rationale and anticipated benefits of bed rests, diagnostic tests (nonstress test [NST], contraction stress test [CST], ultrasonography. Explain diagnostic procedures	Monitor fetal and placental status. NST records fetal heart rate response to activity. CST shows fetal response to imposed stress of contractions. Ultrasonography allows evaluation of fetal size and growth, amni-	Fetal monitor consistently records reactive NST and reassuring pattern on oxytocin challenge test (OCT), i.e., lack of repetitive late decelerations. Ultrasonography reveals normal fetal growth, normal amniotic fluid vol-

(nonstress tests, ultrasonography).	otic fluid volume, and placental grading (including degree of calcification and placental age).	ume, and placenta free of signs of aging.
If monitor reveals fetal tachycardia, bradycardia, late decelerations, loss of baseline variability, provide (1) position change, (2) bolus of IV fluids, and (3) provide oxygen at 6 to 10 L/min by face mask (intrauterine resuscitation).	Increases level of circulating oxygen available to fetus.	FHR returns to normal baseline rate and variability; late decelerations appear.

Continued

NURSING CARE PLAN

CLIENT WITH SEVERE PREGNANCY-INDUCED HYPERTENSION—continued

Goals (expected outcomes)	Interventions	Rationale	Evaluation
ALTERED GENERAL TISSUE PERFUSION—RELATED TO VASOSPASM, HYPERTENSION, AND EDEMA			
Client will experience no alteration in thought processes, blurred vision, increased CNS irritability.	Encourage bedrest in left lateral position.	Promotes increased circulatory volume, renal flow, and diuresis.	Reports no episodes of visual disturbances or altered sensorium. Deep tendon reflexes (DTRs) are normal.
FLUID VOLUME DEFICIT (1)—RELATED TO LOSS OF INTRAVASCULAR FLUID TO EXTRAVASCULAR SPACES			
Client will re-establish normal fluid distribution between intravascular and extravascular compartments.	Encourage high protein intake; reduce intake of foods and fluids that are high in sodium; 6 g sodium allowed per day.	Replaces protein lost in the urine; increases serum albumins; restores normal blood osmolality.	Urine tests negative for protein; edema subsiding; BP and DTRs are within normal limits.

ASSESSMENT

FOCUS ASSESSMENT—HELLP

Estimate number of weeks' gestation.

Note complaints of nausea and upper abdominal discomfort (epigastric pain).

Review findings of diagnostic studies: AST, platelet count, total
bilirubin, hemoglobin and hematocrit, blood glucose, uric acid
level.

Monitor closely vital signs, fetal heart rate, intake and output, results of nonstress testing.

Observe for signs of bleeding, fetal distress, labor, severe preeclampsia.

Elicit information describing perception of self.

Explore nonverbal indicators of emotional status, e.g., affect, mood,
appearance, irritability, inability to concentrate, sleep patterns.

Identify expectations of pregnancy outcome.

Determine individual teaching or learning needs.

Observe family interactions.

CHANGES IN LABORATORY DATA WITH HELLP SYNDROME

Test	Result in healthy pregnancy	Result with HELLP syndrome
Liver Function Tests		
AST	4-20 (1 U/L)	Increased
ALT	3-21 (1 U/L)	Increased
Other Laboratory Values		
Platelets	150,000-400,000/mm³	Decreased
PT	10.2-13.8 sec	Unchanged
PTT	20-31 sec	Unchanged
Fibrinogen	150-400 mg/dl	Increased
Clotting time	Normal	Normal
Total bilirubin	0.2-0.9 mg/dl	Increased
Burr cells	Absent	Present

Adapted from Poole JH: Matern Child Nurs J 13: 432-437, November/
December 1988.

ASSESSMENT

FOCUS ASSESSMENT—PROLONGED PREGNANCY

Monitor closely vital signs, fetal heart rate, results of nonstress tests
and contraction stress tests.

Elicit information regarding self-image.

Explore nonverbal indicators of emotional status, e.g., affect, mood,
appearance, inability to concentrate, sleep patterns.

ASSESSMENT

FOCUS ASSESSMENT—STD

Explore history of past STD and treatment.

Observe for signs of substance abuse. Elicit history as possible.

Elicit information regarding sexual partner(s).

Screen for specific STD (e.g., serologic test for syphilis; culture for
gonorrhea)

Determine level of discomfort (may use a 0 to 10 rating scale to
measure pain)

Observe response to diagnosis.

Elicit information describing perception of self.

Note nonverbal signs of emotional distress (e.g., hostility, inability
to concentrate, withdrawal).

Determine past patterns of coping with crisis.

Identify current support system.

ASSESSMENT

FOCUS ASSESSMENT—HEPATITIS

Note complaints of anorexia, fatigue, nausea, right abdominal discomfort.

Observe for jaundice.

Closely monitor pregnancy progress (weight gain, vital signs, fundal height).

Closely monitor fetal status (fetal heart rate, results of nonstress
testing).

Identify current individual teaching or learning needs.

SEXUALLY TRANSMITTED DISEASES

Syphilis	Gonorrhea	Chlamydia trachomatis infection	Genital herpes
MANIFESTATION			
Latent stage Diagnosis based on serology *Primary stage* Classic lesions called chancres Deep, painful ulcers on genitalia, lips, or rectal area *Secondary stage* Macular rash over body *Third stage* Neurologic symptoms	Nonspecific vaginal discharge	Becoming the most dominant sexually transmitted disease in United States. Cervical infection; sometimes urinary tract infection Vaginal ulcers, cervicitis	1%-2% incidence in pregnant women Painful vesicles in area of vulva and perineum Flu-like symptoms May have inguinal adenopathy
CAUSE			
Treponema pallidum Affects socioeconomically disadvantaged	Gram-negative coccus, neisseria gonorrhoeae Affects mucous membrane of symptomatic carrier (5%-10%)	*Chlamydia trachomatis*	Herpes Type II

Continued

SEXUALLY TRANSMITTED DISEASES—continued

	Syphilis	Gonorrhea	Chlamydia trachomatis infection	Genital herpes
DIAGNOSIS	Positive serology (RPR, VDRL)	Gram-negative coccus, N. gonorrhoeae	Smear and stain examined microscopically Antibody titer (not always accurate) Papanicolaou smear (not specific)	Cytologic smears: reveal large multinucleate cells with eosinophilic inclusion bodies Papanicolaou smear
PROGNOSIS	If detected and treated, no danger to fetus Contagious in all stages Transmitted to fetus through placenta after 18th wk of pregnancy	Risk of permanent injury to infant's eye at birth Can cause serious postpartum infection (pelvic inflammatory disease)	Preterm labor Endometritis postpartum Conjunctivitis in infant with use of tetracycline or erythromycin ophthalmic ointment; *also* pneumonia	Abortion in early pregnancy Preterm labor Microcephaly, microophthalmia in infant Fetus delivered through active lesions has 50% chance of developing
MEDICAL MANAGEMENT	Penicillin G (benzathine) Penicillin G or penicillin G procaine	Single injection of aqueous procaine penicillin	Erythromycin, 500 mg q.i.d. × 7 days	Disseminated herpesvirus infection

Listeriosis	HIV/AIDS	Candidiasis	Trichomonas vaginalis
		cillin preceded by 1 g of probenecid orally	Topical acyclovir Oral acyclovir if taken 4-6 mo, prevents or reduces frequency, duration and severity of recurrence
		Male simultaneously treated with tetracycline	

Erythromycin if allergic to penicillin

Infection may recur (must treat sexual partner also)

Follow client and infant by postpartum serology

Unaffected infant will have positive test if mother is positive

Listeriosis	HIV/AIDS	Candidiasis	Trichomonas vaginalis
MANIFESTATION			
Possible fever of unknown origin	*Early* Initially asymptomatic	Present in 20%-25% of pregnant women	Present in approximately 20% of pregnant women (many asymptomatic)
	More advanced Termed AIDS-related complex *Lymph adenopathy* Severe immune deficiency	Especially prevalent in diabetic pregnant women	
	Full-blown AIDS Pneumocystis carinii pneumonia, Kaposi's sarcoma, and other severe sexually transmitted infections	Increased incidence in pregnant women taking antibiotics or steroids	

Continued

SEXUALLY TRANSMITTED DISEASES—continued

Listeriosis	HIV/AIDS	Candidiasis	Trichomonas vaginalis
MANIFESTATION—cont'd			
		Thick, white, cottage cheese-like appearance to vaginal discharge Burning and itching	White to gray-green foamy discharge Possible inflammation and irritation of vagina and cervix and vulvitis
CAUSE			
Gram-positive bacillus, Listeria monocytogenes	Human immunodeficiency virus (HIV); also called human T-cell lymphotropic virus (causes loss of immunity)	Candida albicans, a fungus	Trichomonas vaginalis
DIAGNOSIS			
Blood and urine cultures	Serologic studies for detection of HIV detection of HIV antibodies or virus	Microscopic examination of vaginal discharge or vaginal culture (culture takes longer)	Microscopic examination of vaginal discharge

PROGNOSIS

50% mortality rates for infected infants *Early onset* clinical signs at birth—respiratory distress, cyanosis, skin lesions, hypothermia *Late onset* (1-6 wk) Meningitis, causing central nervous system damage	Risk of perinatal transmission: 20%-50% Infants with perinatal infection become ill during first 2 yr of life Eventual death for symptomatic clients Concern that pregnancy accelerates AIDS	Possible acquisition of thrush by fetus during delivery process	Medication used for treatment not used during first half of pregnancy because of possible teratogenic effects

MEDICAL MANAGEMENT

Combination of ampicillin or penicillin with gentamicin		Topical miconazole (Monistat) cream or nystatin vaginal suppositories	Metronidazole (Flagyl) orally or vaginally Oral use is avoided during first trimester because of possible teratogenic effects

NURSING CARE PLAN

CLIENT WITH A SEXUALLY TRANSMITTED DISEASE (STD)

Goals (expected outcomes)	Interventions	Rationale	Evaluation
KNOWLEDGE DEFICIT—REGARDING COMPLICATIONS, TREATMENT, AND PREVENTION OF SEXUALLY TRANSMITTED DISEASES			
Client will verbalize understanding of how to prevent infection. Remain free of sexually transmitted diseases.	Teach client cause, mode of transmission, and rationale for treatment.	Assists in understanding how to practice preventive health.	Client discusses basic facts about STDs. Client's secretions are cultured, or client has necessary test for diagnosis.
OR			
Client will verbalize understanding of the disease and its treatment.			
Client will comply with the recommended therapeutic management.	Teach the warning signs of complications: fever, increased pain, bleeding, urinary retention, adenopathy, infection of fetus and inflammation.	Urges client to seek health care.	Client verbalizes warning signs or complications.
Client will recover from the infection.	Refer sexual partner for appropriate treatment.	Imperative to treat all partners.	Sexual partner(s) seeks and receives treatment.
	Teach how and when to take medication and about side effects.	Ensures that infection is properly treated.	Client verbalizes understanding of how and when to take medication.

	Maximizes treatment.	Client takes all medication.
Emphasize the importance of taking all prescribed medication.		
Explain importance of follow-up care.	Begins preventive health measures.	Client returns for follow-up care.

PAIN—RELATED TO INFLAMMATION, ITCHING, OPEN SORES, INVOLVEMENT OF PELVIC ORGANS

Client will experience relief of symptoms.	Administer medication or analgesics as ordered.	Medication used must be safe for mother and infant.	Client has no verbal complaints of pain or verbalizes intensity of discomfort or pain using rating scale.
		Client takes all medication as given or ordered.
Recommend warm sitz baths three to four times a day for genital pain or discomfort.	Warm heat is very soothing for genital or perinatal pain.	Client states warm moist heat or heating pad relieves pain.
Apply heating pad to client's abdomen (if ordered) for abdominal pain.	Decreases abdominal pain.	
Advise client to wear cotton underwear and loose clothing and leave open sores exposed to air.	Keeps genital area clean and dry, promotes healing.	Genital lesions are dry and healing.
Wear gown (impervious) and gloves when in infected area.	Prevents spread of infection.	Client has no spread of infection.
Teach client importance of personal hygiene.	Decreases chance of spread of infection and secondary infection.	Client verbalizes and demonstrates good feminine hygiene.

Continued

NURSING CARE PLAN

CLIENT WITH A SEXUALLY TRANSMITTED DISEASE (STD)—continued

Goals (expected outcomes)	Interventions	Rationale	Evaluation
SITUATIONAL LOW SELF-ESTEEM—RELATED TO PERSONAL PERCEPTIONS OF THE STIGMA OF SEXUALLY TRANSMITTED DISEASE			
Client will work through emotions and accept the disease and its treatment.	Encourage and assist client to verbalize positive and negative feelings toward self.	Feelings must be explored to have insight and understanding of self.	Client expresses feelings about self.
	Clarify misconceptions.	Client must deal with truth, not misconceptions.	Client calmly verbalizes correct information about infection.
	Encourage client to explore and verbalize feelings about her own sexuality.	Feelings are clarified; normal grieving process occurs.	Client speaks about infection and treatment.
	Encourage expressions of anger.	Feelings must be expressed before they can be dealt with.	Client verbalizes angry feelings about infection.
	Encourage verbalization of understanding of connection between life-style and STD.	Must alter life-style to prevent future infections.	Client verbalizes understanding of life-style changes that are necessary.

Chapter 15

INTRAPARTUM COMPLICATIONS

Throughout the labor and delivery process, the nurse is vigilant in assessing and evaluating the client's progress. When labor and delivery fails to proceed as expected or signs and symptoms indicative of other complications occur, the primary care provider is notified. Management of complications of emergency delivery and uterine tetany, rupture, and inversion as well as amniotic fluid embolism and cord prolapse requires alertness and preparedness.

ASSESSMENT

DO'S AND DON'TS OF EMERGENCY CHILDBIRTH (PRECIPITATE LABOR DISORDER)

Do

Remain calm and confident.

Give clear, positive, repeated directions.

Control the delivery of the infant's head.

Clear the infant's airway.

Dry the infant off.

Hold infant at or slightly above level of introitus.

Place infant next to the mother's skin and cover.

Put the infant to breast (if the newborn can reach).

Wait for the placenta to separate.

Inspect placenta for intactness.

Don't

Put fingers into birth canal.

Force rotation of infant's head after head is delivered.

Put traction on cord or pull on cord.

Allow newborn to get cold.

Push on uterus to try to deliver placenta.

DYSTOCIA

Dystocia means "difficult labor" and is characterized by a labor that is abnormally slow. Abnormalities that cause dystocia include:

1. Uterine factors: may be too weak, short, irregular, or infrequent to cause cervical effacement and dilatation, or expulsive forces, both involuntary and voluntary, are insufficient to cause fetal descent.
2. Pelvic factors: The size and shape of the bony pelvis can interfere with the mechanisms of engagement, descent, and expulsion of the fetus.
3. Fetal factors: excessive fetal size, abnormal presentation or position, or abnormalities of the fetus may prevent entrance or passage through the bony pelvis.
4. Psychologic factors: Maternal factors such as anxiety, lack of preparation, and fear can cause a prolonged labor.
5. Position factors: Maternal position can affect the length of first and second stages of labor. The supine position can cause contraction frequency to increase, but contraction intensity decreases. This position also can cause the heavy pregnant uterus to compress the inferior vena cava and aorta. The results are decreased blood flow to the uterus, potential maternal hypotension, and fetal hypoxia.

DYSFUNCTIONAL LABOR

Dysfunctional labor is abnormal uterine contraction patterns. Any of the following can cause dysfunctional labor: (1) premature rupture of the membranes before the onset of labor, (2) analgesia or anesthesia given during the latent phase, (3) overdistention of the uterus (multiple pregnancy, large fetus, or polyhydramnios), (4) grand multiparity, (5) cephalopelvic disproportion, (6) false labor, or (7) uterine abnormalities.

Uterine dysfunction can result in maternal exhaustion and dehydration. Risk for intrauterine infection increases if there is accompanying prolonged rupture of membranes. Maternal hemorrhage from uterine atony after delivery is another complication.

There are five categories or classifications of dysfunctional labor patterns: hypertonic labor, hypotonic labor, uterine tetany, arrest disorders, and precipitous labor.

FOCUS ASSESSMENT—DYSFUNCTIONAL LABOR

Monitor vital signs and fetal heart rate closely.

Note frequency, duration, strength, and interval between contractions.

Identify response to pain.

Monitor intake and output.

Determine current knowledge level regarding condition, implications, and management.

Explore nonverbal indicators of emotional status, e.g., irritability, inability to concentrate, withdrawal.

Explore individual concerns.

Nursing Care Plan

Client with Dysfunctional Labor

Goals (expected outcomes)	Interventions	Rationale	Evaluation
POTENTIAL FOR INFECTION (MATERNAL)—RELATED TO PROLONGED RUPTURE OF MEMBRANES			
Client will experience a progressive labor without an infection.	Record temperature and pulse every 2 hours after rupture of membranes (ROM).	Identifies early signs of infection.	Temperature and pulse normal.
	Keep perineum clean and as dry as possible.	Minimizes or prevents contamination from wet bed.	Client remains free of infection.
	Minimize frequency of vaginal exam.	Reduces the risk for vaginal infection.	Progress is assessed by assessing contractions and response to labor.
	Cleanse perineal area after exams.	Keeps perineal area clean, dry and free of infection.	Perineal care given and taught to client. No signs of infection seen.
	Wash hands before and after client care.	Protects client and self from risk of infection.	Client is free of infection.
POTENTIAL ALTERED UTEROPLACENTAL PERFUSION—RELATED TO HYPERSTIMULATION OF THE UTERUS			
Client will have a progressive labor without hyperstimulation and the fetus will be free of distress.	Run monitor strip on fetus to determine baseline FHR before starting oxytocin infusion.	Ensures fetal heart rate pattern is reassuring.	Baseline fetal heart pattern is normal.

Ensure that physician is readily available while oxytocin infusion is used.	Is available for emergency delivery if there is fetal intolerance to oxytocin.	Physician is present in the hospital.
Always piggyback oxytocin solution into mainline IV line (in port closest to client).	Quickly halts drug absorption and reduces drug-related stimulation of contractions.	Infusion is started with oxytocin piggybacked into mainline.
Increase rate of oxytocin as ordered to elicit effective uterine contractions; discontinue if contractions occur more often than every 2 minutes and last longer than 60 seconds.	Establishes effective uterine contractions; minimizes risk of decreased uteroplacental perfusion and fetal hypoxia.	Monitor records normal pattern of contractions. Labor progresses at normal rate.
Clients with external monitor: note and record uterine response to oxytocin as identified by palpation, i.e., frequency, duration, intensity of contractions, and resting tone.	Distinguishes normal labor pattern from hypertonic pattern and frequency.	Client's labor progresses at normal rate without hypotonic or hypertonic contractions.

Continued

NURSING CARE PLAN

CLIENT WITH DYSFUNCTIONAL LABOR—continued

Goals (expected outcomes)	Interventions	Rationale	Evaluation
POTENTIAL ALTERED UTEROPLACENTAL PERFUSION—RELATED TO HYPERSTIMULATION OF THE UTERUS—cont'd			
	With internal monitor: record intrauterine resting tone and intensity.	Identifies presence of normal vs. hypertonic vs. hypotonic contractions.	Normal contraction pattern is occurring.
	Change position every 30 minutes from sitting upright vs. up and walking (if presenting part well engaged).	Offers more positions for fetal descent and internal rotation to anterior.	Normal patterns of fetal descent in anterior position.
	Encourage client to avoid supine position.	Avoids aortocaval compression and interruption of blood flow to uterus and through placenta.	Client has normal blood pressure; fetal monitor records normal baseline FHR; fetus is reactive with good baseline variability and reassuring fetal heart patterns.
	Encourage emptying bladder every 2 hours.	Full bladder may impede labor failure to progress.	Client voids and empties bladder every 2 hours.
	Record intake and output.	Adequate circulatory vol-	Client takes ice chips and

	Initiate intrauterine resuscitation if there is hyperstimulation or a nonreassuring pattern noted:	ume maintains cardiac output and adequate uteroplacental perfusion.	voids clear urine every 2 hours.
		Improves uteroplacental blood flow.	Normal contraction pattern; fetus has normal baseline FHR, reactivity, variability, and no periodic fetal heart tones.
	Turn off oxytocin.	Decreases stimulation of uterine activity.	
	Turn to side.	Prevents aortocaval compression.	
	Speed up mainline infusion.	Increases blood flow to heart and therefore to uterus, placenta, and to baby.	
	Give oxygen 6-8 L/m by tight face mask.	Assists maternal oxygenation.	
	Report and record.	Documents nursing care.	
FLUID VOLUME DEFICIT—RELATED TO PROLONGED LABOR AND RESTRICTED FLUID INTAKE			
Client will exhibit normal state of hydration.	Offer ice chips.	Decreases thirst and dryness of mouth which accompanies labor.	Client states ice quenches her thirst and adds to her comfort.
	Check urine for acetone.	Identifies signs of dehydration.	Urine is negative for acetone.

Continued

Nursing Care Plan

Client with Dysfunctional Labor—continued

Goals (expected outcomes)	Interventions	Rationale	Evaluation
FLUID VOLUME DEFICIT—RELATED TO PROLONGED LABOR AND RESTRICTED FLUID INTAKE—cont'd			
	Encourage to void about every 2 hours.	Assesses hydration.	Client voids clear, straw- or amber-colored urine every 2 hours.
	Give IV fluids as ordered.	Ensures hydration.	Client retains normal fluid volume as evidenced by vital signs and intake-output ratio.
—RELATED TO UTERINE CONTRACTIONS			
Client will experience relief of pain; verbalize sense of control of situation, and make informed choice among available alternatives.	Review comfort measures and pain relieving techniques.	Provides choices for pain relief and enables selection of method appropriate to individual needs and desires.	Client uses breathing and relaxation techniques very effectively.
	Assist with relaxation techniques.	Relaxation decreases perception of pain and increases the efficacy of analgesia/anesthesia.	Client relaxes easily; states pain is tolerable.
	Explain options for pain re-	Involves client in decision	Client verbalizes under-

lief (analgesic, anesthesia).	making regarding analgesia/anesthesia.	standing of options available for pain relief and remains calm and responds to nursing interventions.
Encourage mother and father and provide positive feedback.	Parents need encouragement and praise for their efforts; supports positive self-image and coping abilities.	Client and husband effectively work together and display no evidence of panic and discouragement.
Encourage client to utilize alternate positions to assist progress.	Upright or left lateral and change of position every 30 minutes often will improve contraction effectiveness.	Client remains relaxed with position changes. Fetal monitor records normal baseline FHR.
Record and report characteristics of uterine contractions, i.e., frequency, duration, intensity, and resting tone.	Determines efficient vs. incoordinate contractions.	Contractions are effective and there is good oxygenation of fetus.

ANXIETY—RELATED TO LACK OF LABOR PROGRESS

Client's feelings of anxiety will be allayed by explanation.	Listen, take time to touch, and show concern.	Helps client to feel situation is under control and people are concerned and want to help.	Client states she is more relaxed.

Continued

NURSING CARE PLAN

CLIENT WITH DYSFUNCTIONAL LABOR—continued

Goals (expected outcomes)	Interventions	Rationale	Evaluation
ANXIETY—RELATED TO LACK OF LABOR PROGRESS—cont'd			
	Explain reasons for dysfunctional labor and what plan of care will be.	Fear of unknown is greater than having some understanding of what is happening.	Client verbalizes understanding of dysfunctional labor and management.
KNOWLEDGE DEFICIT—RELATED TO DYSFUNCTIONAL LABOR AND INTRAVENOUS OXYTOCIN FOR AUGMENTATION OF LABOR			
Client and family will verbalize understanding of reason for oxytocic augmentation and effects expected.	Reinforce physician's explanations of oxytocin augmentation of labor.	Increases understanding of procedure; reduces anxiety and fear; increases cooperation.	Couple reports they are less fearful and anxious.
	Explain how procedure will be done.	Increases knowledge and allays fear of unknown.	Couple verbalizes understanding and readiness to begin.
	Explain what to expect from oxytocin drip.	Prepares for contractions that can effect progress.	Couple verbalizes their desire for labor to progress and their infant to be born.

Chapter 16

POSTPARTUM COMPLICATIONS

Post partum is a time of increased physiologic and psychologic stress for the family as the mother's body returns to a nonpregnant state and new family roles are assumed. Many complications can occur during the postpartum period, but only three are serious or life-threatening: hemorrhage, infection, and embolism. The nurse must be familiar with the normal anatomy and physiology of the puerperium to identify the deviations from normal as soon as possible. All information collected about the client from prenatal visits, during admission, and through labor and delivery must be reviewed to identify risk factors that would produce complications.

HEMORRHAGIC COMPLICATIONS

ASSESSMENT

CONDITIONS PREDISPOSING FOR POSTPARTUM HEMORRHAGE*

Antedating pregnancy	Arising during pregnancy and labor
Previous postpartum hemorrhage	Placenta previa
Grand multiparity	Abruptio placentae
Fibroids	Multiple pregnancy
Idiopathic thrombocytopenia purpura	Polyhydramnios
Von Willebrand's disease	Precipitate labor
Leukemia	Prolonged labor
	Chorioamnionitis
	Forceps delivery
	Cesarean section
	General anesthesia
	Mismanagement of third stage of labor
	Acute coagulation defect

---

*From Cavanaugh D et al: Obstetric Emergencies, 3rd ed. New York, Harper & Row, 1982.

SIGNS AND SYMPTOMS OF SHOCK

	Presenting signs and symptoms	
Factor	**Hypovolemic shock**	**Septic shock**
Pulse	Tachycardia: weak, thready pulse	Tachycardia: rebounding pulse, palpitations
Blood pressure	Hypotension: anxious, restless	Hypotension: faint, dizzy
Tissue perfusion	Decreased: cold clammy skin, pale, cyanotic nail beds, flat neck veins	Cerebral ischemia: anxiety, apprehension, disorientation, stupor
Urinary output	Oliguria: 50 ml/hr; urinary sodium—80 mEq/L	Polyuria: 125 ml/hr; urinary sodium—10mEq/L

SHOCK

Perineum: obvious bleeding
Fundus: firm vs. boggy, fundal height
Vital signs
　Respirations: tachypnea, shallow, irregular, air hunger
　Pulse: tachycardia, weak, thready, irregular
　Blood pressure: hypotensive, dizziness, faintness
Skin: cool, moist, pale, cold, clammy, cyanosis of lips and fingernails, capillar refill
Urinary output: decreasing, <30 ml/hr
Level of consciousness: oriented, mental cloudiness, increasing restlessness, lethargy
Psychologic status: anxious
Laboratory values
　CBC
　Electrolytes (including blood urea nitrogen and creatinine)
　Blood gases
　Coagulation profile
　Urinalysis
　Type and crossmatch

Sample Narrative Charting: Complains of being dizzy. "I feel like I'm going to faint." Lying on stretcher in pool of blood, which has soaked through two maxi sanitary pads as well as underpad. Fundus is boggy and does not firm with massage. Asked another nurse to get physician STAT. Blood pressure is 60/0, pulse is 120, weak, and thready, respirations are 28 and shallow. Skin is cold and clammy and diaphoretic. Placed in Trendelenburg position and intravenous of Ringer's lactate started in left forearm. Oxygen at 8 L per mask started. Bleeding still profuse. Methergine 0.2 mg given IV push as ordered.

DEGREE OF HEMORRHAGE

Severity	Signs and symptoms	Reduction in blood volume
Mild	Uterine consistency firm or boggy	15%-20% (750-1250 ml)
	Bleeding from vaginal or cervical lacerations	
	Slight or no decrease in blood pressure (1500 ml of blood can be lost before significant drop in blood pressure occurs	
	Minimum tachycardia	
	Mild evidence of vasoconstriction, with cool hands and feet	
Moderate	Atonic uterus decreased pulse pressure	25%-35% (1250-1750 ml)
	Systolic pressure 90-100 mm Hg	
	Tachycardia (100-120 bpm)	
	Restlessness	
	Sweating	
	Pallor	
	Oliguria	
Severe	Atonic uterus	Up to 50% (2500 ml)
	Systolic pressure decreased to 60 mm Hg and frequently unobtainable by cuff	
	Tachycardia >120 bpm	
	Mental stupor	
	Extreme pallor	
	Cold extremities	
	Anuria	

Nursing Care Plan

Client With the Complications of Hemorrhage and Shock

Goals

ALTERATION IN CARDIAC OUTPUT—RELATED TO HYPOVOLEMIA
ALTERATION IN TISSUE PERFUSION—RELATED TO DECREASED BLOOD VOLUME SECONDARY TO HEMORRHAGE AND SHOCK

(expected outcomes)	Interventions	Rationale	Evaluation
Client will maintain adequate cardiac output and tissue perfusion.	Maintain bed rest in modified Trendelenburg position.	Increases venous blood return to heart.	Blood pressure is stable and comparable to values occurring before bleeding.
	Record vital signs every 15 min or more (often depending on severity of blood loss and shock); report significant changes promptly.	Assists in determining physiologic response to blood loss.	All vital signs are in range established before bleeding.
	Evaluate amount of blood loss by counting and weighing pads and linen. Contact primary health care provider immediately in case of hemorrhage.	Provides more objective information than visual evaluation.	Blood loss is minimal.
	Ensure IV is patent or get order for placement of an IV line. Use lactated Ringer's solution or normal saline so-	Orders should be received and implemented quickly to prevent further complications.	Fluid volume is maintained.

lution to replace volume initially.		
Ensure bladder emptying; if unsure, request order for indwelling catheter.	Hypovolemia reduces kidney perfusion and decreases urinary output.	Kidney perfusion is stable as evidenced by 50-100 ml urinary output hourly.
Check for central vs. peripheral cyanosis, paleness, skin tugor, and diaphoresis.	Determines general perfusion status, i.e., central to peripheral.	Skin is pink centrally and peripherally and is warm and dry.
Administer blood plasma or volume expander as ordered.	Replaces circulating volume, increases blood return to heart, and increases perfusion to all organs.	Blood pressure and other vital signs are within normal limits, and urinary output is 50-100 ml/hr.
Keep client and family informed.	Allays some anxiety.	Client and family verbalize they are no longer anxious.
Administer oxygen by face mask at 6-8 L/min.	Increases oxygenation.	Client's color is pink, she reports no dizziness, and no other signs of shock are present.

Continued

NURSING CARE PLAN

CLIENT WITH THE COMPLICATIONS OF HEMORRHAGE AND SHOCK—continued

Goals (expected outcomes)	Interventions	Rationale	Evaluation
ANXIETY—RELATED TO THE PHYSIOLOGIC CRISIS OF HEMORRHAGE			
Client will express concerns and fears instead of holding them in and becoming very anxious.	Convey attitude of confidence and calm.	Client needs to feel nurse and physician are confident about her care (they are in control of the situation at hand).	Client verbalizes confidence in her care.
	Explain all care.	Helps decrease some anxiety; increases confidence in care.	Client understands much of what is being done for her and conveys confidence in her care.
	Maintain atmosphere of quiet and calm.	Helps maintain calmness in client.	Client and family remain calm.
	Keep client informed of status. Give realistic, factual information about her status.	Directs worry at reality instead of fantasized problems. Helps maintain client's calmness and confidence.	Worry is properly directed at what is real.

Allow support person(s) to stay with client as much as possible.	Allays some worries and fears of support person(s).	Support person(s) is calm and cooperative.
Administer medications as ordered for pain.	Maintains comfort.	Client states she is comfortable.
Remain with client.	Provides supportive care and builds relationship.	Client responds to nursing assurance and support.
Encourage expression of feelings, asking of questions.	Helps nurse to anticipate client's worries and fears and to allay them when possible.	Atmosphere is conducive to open communication and assistance.
Support positive coping mechanisms of client, family, or support person(s).	Facilitates effective coping with stress.	Client and support person are coping effectively.
Provide information about infant.	Promotes bonding.	Client talks about infant.

Continued

NURSING CARE PLAN

CLIENT WITH THE COMPLICATIONS OF HEMORRHAGE AND SHOCK—continued

Goals (expected outcomes)	Interventions	Rationale	Evaluation
KNOWLEDGE DEFICIT—REGARDING CAUSE OF POSTPARTUM HEMORRHAGE AND ITS MANAGEMENT			
Client will verbalize understanding of postpartum hemorrhage, how it is managed, and follow-up care.	Explain why postpartum hemorrhage occurs.	Increases understanding of the process.	Client asks questions and discusses how postpartum hemorrhage affects unfulfilled birth plans.
	Encourage questions about care, procedures, and overall management.	Increases understanding of care given.	Client is compliant with care, asks questions easily.
	Explain effects of oxytocic drugs, particularly stimulation of contractions, which may cause cramping, and involution (to decrease bleeding).	Promotes understanding of drug effects so there is no concern or worry about stimulated contractions.	Client verbalizes understanding of effects of oxytocic medications.
	Explain need for continued observation and assessment to ensure normal involution vs. further bleeding.	Ensures risk of bleeding is diminishing.	Client experiences normal involution.

ASSESSMENT—POSTPARTUM GENITAL TRACT INFECTION

TYPES OF POSTPARTUM GENITAL TRACT INFECTIONS

Type of infection	Etiology	Signs and symptoms	Treatment
Perineal and vulvar lesions	Bacterial invasion of episiotomy, laceration, traumatized tissue	Fever, localized pain Edema, erythema; seropurulent discharge from lesion; usually occurs after day 5	Antibiotics Removal of stitches and promotion of drainage, sitz baths, perineal heat lamp, analgesics
Endometritis	Bacterial invasion of placental site or entire endometrium	Fever of approximately 38.4°C (101°F), chills, rapid pulse, usually occurs within 48 hr of delivery Malaise, headache, backache, loss of appetite, cramps Relaxed, tender uterus with foul-smelling discharge, dark or profuse lochia	Antibiotics, ergonovine Fowler's position to promote drainage, hydration

Continued

ASSESSMENT—POSTPARTUM GENITAL TRACT INFECTION

TYPES OF POSTPARTUM GENITAL TRACT INFECTIONS—continued

Type of infection	Etiology	Signs and symptoms	Treatment
Pelvic cellulitis or parametritis	Bacterial invasion by way of lymphatics to tissue surrounding uterus (often following endometritis)	Fever, chills Pain and tenderness of lower abdomen, edema Signs of endometritis may be present also	Antibiotics Hydration, blood transfusion for dropping hemoglobin Bed rest, analgesics
Peritonitis	Spread of infection to peritoneum, local or generalized	High fever, rapid pulse Severe abdominal pain Vomiting, restlessness Distention	Antibiotics, analgesics, sedatives Bed rest, hydration, blood transfusion, oxygen, IV fluids
Salpingitis and oophoritis	Spread of infection to fallopian tubes and ovaries	Lower abdominal pain Temperature elevation, tachycardia Nausea and vomiting	Antibiotics, analgesics, sedatives, antipyretics Hydration, IV fluids

Assessment—Cystitis and Pyelonephritis

Urinary Tract Infection

Dysuria
Frequency
Urgency
Urinary retention; inability to empty bladder completely
Marked tenderness and discomfort over bladder area
Low-grade fever
Leukocytosis noted in catheterized urine specimen

Specific to Pyelonephritis
Chills
Elevated temperature
Flank pain (on side of affected kidney)

CLIENT SELF-CARE EDUCATION: POSTPARTUM CYSTITIS AND PYELONEPHRITIS

Action	Rationale
1. Empty bladder as soon as possible after delivery (within 6–8 hr).	1. Retention of residual urine, bladder trauma during delivery, and catheterization (if done) increase risk for bladder infection.
2. Use helpful tips to encourage voiding: a. Straddle toilet instead of sitting. b. Run water in sink. c. Squirt warm water over perineum with peri-bottle. d. Take an analgesic a few minutes before trying to void. e. Sit in sitz bath to void.	2. Promotes relaxation and reduces discomfort of voiding.
3. Spend time after each voiding to make sure bladder is empty.	3. Ensures bladder emptying and prevents urinary retention and bladder distention.
4. Wash hands after voiding.	4. Decreases contamination from hands.

5. Drink plenty of fluids even if no voiding problems exist.
6. Measure urine during first few voidings.
7. If the following symptoms occur, report them to primary care provider:
   a. Pain with urination
   b. Frequency
   c. Urgency
   d. Inability to empty bladder
   e. Tenderness or discomfort over bladder area
   f. Low-grade fever
8. Report chills, fever, and flank pain *IMMEDIATELY* to primary care provider.
9. Take all prescribed medications *exactly* as instructed.
10. Keep follow-up health care appointments.

5. Promotes diuresis of increased circulatory volume.
6. Ensures bladder is emptying and prevents urinary retention.
7. Symptoms require laboratory follow-up study so treatment can be initiated.
8. Prompt reporting initiates prompt intervention.
9. Antibiotics are ineffective unless the full course is taken.
10. Ensures that treatment is promptly rendered.

ASSESSMENT

PREGNANCY RISK FACTORS FOR THROMBOEMBOLIC CONDITIONS

Maternal age greater than 35 yr
Obesity
Immobilization
Cardiopulmonary disease
Diabetes mellitus
Previous history of thromboembolism
Traumatic delivery

FOCUS ASSESSMENT—THROMBOEMBOLIC CONDITIONS

Examine for Homans' sign, tenderness over involved vein.

Monitor vital signs closely.

Inspect for signs of complications of therapy (e.g., bleeding gums, easy bruising, return of lochial rubra).

Be alert to signs of pulmonary embolus (e.g., severe chest pain, dyspnea, diaphoresis).

Review diagnostic studies (e.g., Lee-White clotting time, prothrombin time [PT], partial thromboplastin time [PTT]).

Explore client's nonverbal indicators of emotional stress and coping (e.g., irritability, inability to concentrate, withdrawal).

Explore individual concerns.

Determine client's current level of knowledge regarding disorder, implications, and therapy.

Identify individual learning needs.

NURSING CARE PLAN

CLIENT WITH THROMBOEMBOLIC CONDITION

Goals (expected outcomes)	Interventions	Rationale	Evaluation
POTENTIAL FOR PAIN—RELATED TO VENOUS THROMBOSIS OR SUPERFICIAL THROMBOPHLEBITIS			
The client will regain health, be free from complications (pulmonary embolism) of thromboembolic condition, and express understanding of disease process and ways to minimize future development.	Maintain bed rest for client, with affected leg elevated for 5-7 days or until symptoms are clear.	Reduces tension on vein, increases venous return of blood to heart, and decreases edema.	Edema is decreasing; leg is warm and color is good.
	Apply proper fitting antiembolic stocking and apply continuous moist heat to leg.	Speeds resolution of inflammation and pain.	Client states has less pain; redness and warmth (heat) of skin have lessened.
	Measure thighs and calves daily.	Assesses resolution of edema by measuring calf circumference (2 cm difference is significant).	Edema is decreasing with <2 cm difference in circumferences of calves and thighs.
	Provide analgesia for pain.	Decreases pain.	Client verbalizes that pain has lessened.

Continued

Nursing Care Plan

CLIENT WITH THROMBOEMBOLIC CONDITION—continued

Goals (expected outcomes)	Interventions	Rationale	Evaluation
POTENTIAL FOR PAIN—RELATED TO VENOUS THROMBOSIS OR SUPERFICIAL THROMBOPHLEBITIS—cont'd			
	Instruct client to report all pain, especially chest pain, and shortness of breath.	Symptoms may indicate presence of embolus that may lodge in heart or lungs.	Client states no chest pain or shortness of breath is experienced.
ALTERATION IN TISSUE PERFUSION: PERIPHERAL—RELATED TO VENOUS THROMBOSIS			
Client will maintain adequate peripheral circulation.	Assess peripheral circulation every 4 hr (palpable pulse, skin temperature, color, and edema); may check Homan's sign (calf pain when leg extended and foot dorsiflexed).	Ensures peripheral circulation is maintained.	Client has strong palpable pulses in all extremities and maintains good skin color.
	Instruct client to avoid use of knee gatch on bed and pillow under knees.	Avoids further pressure on vessels, which would inhibit venous return to heart.	Venous circulation is maintained as evidenced by strong palpable pulses and good skin color.

Instruct client to avoid massaging and rubbing legs.	Avoids risk of dislodging thrombus.	Client states she understands importance of avoiding massage, rubbing legs.
Change client's position every 2 hr and instruct her about and assist her with active and passive range of joint motion exercises as ordered.	Increases circulation and avoids excessive pressure on dependent areas.	Client changes position at least every 2 hr. Her skin color is good; no dependent areas are reddened or broken down.
Apply antiembolic stockings	Increases circulation.	Circulation is maintained as evidenced by palpable peripheral pulses.
Remove antiembolic stockings once every 8 hr for 15 min; assess skin carefully for signs of breakdown.	Ensures that all skin surfaces are intact.	All skin surfaces are intact, with no visible breakdown or loss of skin integrity.
Encourage intake of nutritional diet and fluids.	Provides cellular nutrition and circulating blood volume.	All skin surfaces have good color and are intact; all peripheral pulses are strong by palpation.

Continued

NURSING CARE PLAN

CLIENT WITH THROMBOEMBOLIC CONDITION—continued

Goals (expected outcomes)	Interventions	Rationale	Evaluation
POTENTIAL FOR INJURY (BLEEDING)—RELATED TO SIDE EFFECTS OF FIBRINOLYTIC OR ANTICOAGULANT THERAPY			
Client will maintain all coagulation studies within acceptable limits and display no signs of bleeding.	Administer anticoagulants as ordered.	Prevents development of thrombosis and dissolves formed emboli.	Client's coagulation studies reveal improvement.
	Check client for bleeding gums, hematuria, epistaxis, petechiae, gastrointestinal or rectal bleeding.	Use of anticoagulants may cause bleeding at any vulnerable body site.	No bleeding is noted at any body site.
	Check laboratory results for prolonged prothrombin and clotting times.	Determines from laboratory results if bleeding is anticipated.	Coagulation studies are in acceptable limits.
KNOWLEDGE DEFICIT—REGARDING THROMBOEMBOLIC CONDITION, ITS MANAGEMENT, AND AVOIDANCE OF ITS RECURRENCE			
Client will be compliant with all care and will ask questions and verbalize knowledge about her care and medi-	Teach client about venous stasis and its relationship to potential embolus formation (e.g., sitting with legs crossed, massaging legs, immobility, pres-	Avoids measures that cause stasis and thrombus formation.	Client verbalizes understanding of stasis and how to avoid it.

cation, about precautionary measures to avoid venous stasis and bleeding, about exercises, and about signs and symptoms that would require reporting to and seeing the primary health care provider.		
Teach client how to apply elastic (antiembolic) stockings (be sure she knows to avoid all constrictive clothing) and how to perform range of joint motion exercises.	Increases circulation and avoids stasis.	Client demonstrates application of elastic stockings and performance of range of motion exercises.
Teach early signs of thrombosis and thrombophlebitis (stiffness, soreness, swelling, redness over affected area).	Increases understanding of signs and symptoms of thromboembolic condition and complications.	Client verbalizes signs and symptoms to monitor and to report to primary health care provider.
Explain schedule, dosage, action, and side effects of prescribed medications.	Enhances understanding of drug therapy (especially anticoagulant therapy).	Client verbalizes schedule, dosage, actions, and side effects of drugs.

Continued

NURSING CARE PLAN

CLIENT WITH THROMBOEMBOLIC CONDITION—continued

Goals (expected outcomes)	Interventions	Rationale	Evaluation
KNOWLEDGE DEFICIT—REGARDING THROMBOEMBOLIC CONDITION, ITS MANAGEMENT, AND AVOIDANCE OF ITS RECURRENCE—cont'd			
	Suggest guidelines (e.g., use soft toothbrush, avoid going barefoot, wear gloves to do cleaning) to avoid hazards that could cause bleeding during anticoagulant therapy in hospital and after discharge.	Avoids side effects of bleeding during anticoagulant therapy.	Client begins practices that will avoid injury that could cause bleeding.
	Instruct client to tell all other health care providers (e.g., dentist), she is receiving anticoagulant therapy.	Ensures avoidance of risks that could cause bleeding.	Client notes other health care providers who may be used during time of anticoagulant therapy.
	Teach client about stasis, thromboembolic condition, and managment at times when significant others are available to receive teaching and ask questions.	Increases understanding of venous stasis, thromboemoblic condition, and its management.	Client and her family verbalize understanding of thromboembolic condition; their responses to questions verify their knowledge.

NEWBORN COMPLICATIONS

Chapter 17

THE NEONATE WITH DEVELOPMENTAL OR ACQUIRED DISORDERS

The etiology of birth defects is not completely understood. Because birth defects are so numerous and varied, this chapter presents selected disorders—those more commonly seen that are apparent at birth or soon thereafter. The care of these infants and their parents presents a challenge to the nurse who must give competent, complex nursing care to the infants as well as help parents cope with their feelings of disappointment and despair.

ASSESSMENT AND INTERVENTION

CONGENITAL ABNORMALITY NURSING CARE SUMMARY

Congenital abnormality	Assessment	Nursing interventions in the early neonatal period	Therapeutic management
Cleft lip and cleft palate	May occur separately, bilaterally or unilaterally Occurs in 1:2500 births Cleft lip ranges from slight dimple to wide separation extending to the nasal structures Cleft palate may involve the soft palate alone; can extend along the hard palate and the anterior portions of the maxilla	Encourage parents to hold and touch infant. Provide information about care of infant (see Client Infant Care Education: Feeding Newborn With Cleft Palate).	Establishment of nutrition Avoiding aspiration Early referral to plastic surgeon Long-term: Orthodontic care, speech therapy, hearing evaluation
Tracheoesophageal atresia, type 3, with esophageal fistula	Most common of the esophageal deformities Large amounts of oral secretions Choking on feedings Aspiration of stomach contents through the fistula into the trachea	Perform frequent, careful suctioning. Avoid oral feedings. Keep infant in semi-upright position to avoid reflux of stomach contents into the trachea.	Immediate gastrostomy to reduce risk of reflux of stomach contents into trachea Intravenous (IV) fluids Antibiotics

Continued

ASSESSMENT AND INTERVENTION

CONGENITAL ABNORMALITY NURSING CARE SUMMARY—continued

Congenital abnormality	Assessment	Nursing interventions in the early neonatal period	Therapeutic management
Signs of aspirating pneumonitis: tachypnea, tachycardia, pallor, cyanosis, retractions, rhonchi, decreased breath sounds			Surgical repair to close fistula and join (anastomose) esophagus; segment of colon may be used if esophagus is too short to join
Diaphragmatic hernia	Severe respiratory distress shortly after birth	Place infant in upright position.	Immediate surgical repair
	Protrusion of abdominal contents into chest and compression of lung tissue	Pass nasogastric tube to remove air from stomach.	IV fluids
	Respiratory distress more severe as bowel fills with air during the first hours of life	Administer oxygen.	Antibiotics if infection occurs
		Turn to affected side to permit expansion of unaffected lung.	
Imperforate anus	Inability to take rectal temperature	Observe every infant carefully for passing of first stool, abdominal distention, and	Surgery
	Abdominal distention		May need colostomy until complete repair
	Meconium stools not present		

	Shallow blind, rectal pouch instead of normal anal opening; Possible fistula to bladder, vagina, or urethra	failure to pass rectal thermometer. Report deviations from normal to physician.	
Omphalocele	Protrusion of abdominal contents through umbilical opening; Bowel covered by amniotic membrane, not skin	Immediately cover omphalocele with sterile gauze moistened with warm sterile water. Keep it moist until surgery is performed. Cover it with plastic wrap. Handle infant gently. Protect sac to prevent rupture. Prevent infection by using sterile gloves when providing care.	Nasogastric tube to prevent distention of bowel. If peritoneal cavity not large enough to provide room for intestines, abdominal skin may be used to cover until complete repair. Total IV alimentation may be necessary
Myelomeningocele	Saclike mass containing spinal cord, nerve roots, and meningeal covering; protrudes	Protect lesion from trauma and infection.	Surgical correction early to prevent sepsis

Continued

ASSESSMENT AND INTERVENTION

CONGENITAL ABNORMALITY NURSING CARE SUMMARY—continued

Congenital abnormality	Assessment	Nursing interventions in the early neonatal period	Therapeutic management
	through bony defect in thoracic or lumbar spine (spina bifida) Level of defect determined by neurologic involvement Paralysis of extremities Poor bowel and bladder control Sensory deficits below level of defect Associated with hydrocephalus	Position infant on abdomen or side. Prevent fecal or urinary contamination. Use sterile dressing over sac to prevent rupture and drying. Change position frequently. Observe sac for oozing or pus.	Observation for hydrocephalus IV fluids Antibiotics
Hydrocephalus	Enlargement of cerebral ventricles resulting from abnormal amount of cerebral fluid Enlarging head size Wide separations of suture lines Bulging fontanels Shiny, thin-skinned appearance of forehead, with visible veins Setting-sun appearance of eyes	Protect head from injury. Provide support for head. Measure and record head circumference daily. Observe fontanel for bulging.	Surgical placement of shunt to allow cerebrospinal fluid to circulate

	Signs of increased intracranial pressure Lethargy High-pitched cry Irritability Vomiting Convulsions Transillumination of head indicating translucency (presence of fluid rather than cerebral tissue)	Place sponge-rubber pad under head or using alternating mattress. Change position frequently.	
Down syndrome (trisomy 21, translocation, or mosaicism)	Trisomy 21 type occurs more often in children of women more than 35 years old Found in eary race, color, creed Flat occiput Eyes upslanted with epicanthal folds Protruding tongue Short, broad neck Hypotonic muscles Short limbs Broad, square hands	Support parents by standing by, listening, helping them formulate questions. Call infant by name. Encourage parents to hold and feed infant. Assist parents with feedings. Contact support group.	Frequently diagnosed at birth because of obvious signs When diagnosis suspected, chromosomal analysis is ordered to determine specific cause; information is useful for genetic counseling Information about disorder and prognosis provided by physician Parents referred to appropriate community resources by physician

CONGENITAL HEART DISEASE

Structural heart defects are categorized by two features: (1) the abnormality results in cyanosis and (2) the pulmonary blood flow is increased, normal or decreased.

Cyanotic heart defects

Tetralogy of Fallot
Transposition of Great Vessesl
Hypoplastic Heart Syndrome

Acyanotic heart defects

Patent Ductus Arteriosus
Ventricular Septal Defect
Atrial Septal Defect
Coarctation of the Aorta

ASSESSMENT

SIGNS THAT CAN INDICATE CONGENITAL HEART DEFECTS

Heart murmurs and dysrhythmias
Dyspnea (retractions, grunting,
  nasal flaring)
Tachypnea
Pulmonary edema
Tachycardia
Cyanotic episodes
Central cyanosis
Lethargy
Difficulty in feeding
Failure to gain weight
Absent or unequal pulses

SIGNS OF NEONATAL CONGESTIVE HEART FAILURE

Edema   Diaphoresis
Fatigue   Decreased urinary output
Pallor   Rales

HYPERBILIRUBINEMIA OR PATHOLOGIC JAUNDICE IN THE NEONATE

Physiologic hyperbilirubinemia results from the following: interference in the conjugation of bilirubin; interference in elimination of bilirubin from the body; decrease in the production of the liver enzyme glucuronyl transferase; hemolysis of a large number of RBCs coupled with the shortened life span of the newborn RBCs.

ASSESSMENT

BILIRUBIN LEVELS*

	Term infant (mg)	Preterm infant (mg)
Cord blood	2	—
Mean peak of bilirubin at 60-72 hr	6	Rises more rapidly in preterm infant; jaundice occurs at lower levels
Indication for photo-therapy	12*	10* (lower for smaller infants)
Indication for exchange transfusion	20*	15* (lower for smaller infants)

From Korones SB, Lancaster J: High-risk Newborn Infants. St. Louis, CV Mosby, 1981.

*These values are guides. Variables such as size, age, rapidity of rise of bilirubin level, other test results, and cause of hyperbilirubinemia enter into the physician's decision to initiate therapy.

PATHOLOGIC JAUNDICE OF NEWBORN WITH RH SENSITIZATION

Test	Results
Rh factor	Rh positive
Direct Coombs'	Positive
Total serum bilirubin level in first 24 hr	Elevated >6 mg/dl
Direct (conjugated) serum bilirubin level	More than 1-2 mg/dl
Daily increases in total serum bilirubin level	More than 5 mg/dl/24 hr
Total serum bilirubin level (combination of direct and indirect)	More than 12 mg/dl
Reticulocytes (3%-7%)	>6% after third day of life
Hemoglobin (15-18 g/dl)	Low value suggests anemia

ONGOING ASSESSMENT OF THE NEWBORN FOR JAUNDICE

1. Report jaundice that occurs in the first 24 hr of life or that continues beyond 1 week in the full-term newborn.
2. Press firmly on the skin, especially over bony prominences, i.e., forehead, nose, and sternum.
   a. Jaundice first appears on face and upper body.
   b. After pressure is released, area appears yellow.
3. Observe sclera and oral mucous membrane, especially in dark-skinned infants.
4. Jaundice deepens in color and advances to trunk and extremities as serum bilirubin level rises.
5. Assess newborn for conditions associated with jaundice, i.e., bruising, cephalohematoma, breast-feeding, Rh factor, maternal blood type O.

Nursing Care Plan

BABY WITH HYPERBILIRUBINEMIA

Goals (expected outcome)	Interventions	Rationale	Evaluation
FLUID VOLUME DEFICIT (2)—RELATED TO FLUID LOSS			
Newborn's temperature will remain within normal parameters during phototherapy (36.5°-37°C).	Offer feeding every 3-4 hr.	Adequate fluid intake is 140-200 ml/kg/24 hr. Replaces fluid losses.	Temperature within normal parametes (97°-99° F axillary) Fontanels not depressed Skin not tenting Urinary output >30 ml/kg/24 hr Six diapers moderately saturated in 24 hr Weight loss not <5% in 24 hr Newborn weighing 3200 g—intake is approximately 74-100 ml every 4 hr

Continued

Nursing Care Plan

Baby with Hyperbilirubinemia—continued

Goals (expected outcome)	Interventions	Rationale	Evaluation
POTENTIAL FOR INJURY—RELATED TO HAZARDS OF PHOTOTHERAPY			
Infant will exhibit no signs of redness, edema, or drainage from eyes during phototherapy.	Place eye patches securely over infant's eyes during phototherapy. Evaluate placement at least every 2 hr.	Patches protects eyes from direct, bright lights. Patches may be dislodged during activity and crying. Detects conjunctivitis early.	Eye patches securely in place while infant is under phototherapy No signs of redness, edema, or discharge from eyes
POTENTIAL IMPAIRED SKIN INTEGRITY—RELATED TO EXCORIATION FROM LOOSE STOOLS			
Newborn's skin in genital and rectal areas will remain intact.	Cleanse genital and rectal area gently with warm water and pat dry.	Phototherapy can cause more frequent, loose, green stools as conjugated bilirubin is excreted. Stools may be irritating and cause excoriation in the rectal and genital areas.	Skin free of irritation
ALTERED FAMILY PROCESS			
Newborn will experience periods of social contact with parents or caregiver.	Shut off bili-light and remove eye patches during parent contact and feeding. Encourage parents to	Provides frequent visual stimulation. Promotes parental attachment.	Parents exhibit signs of bonding, e.g., eye contact, cuddling, calling by name

hold and feed, stroke
and touch baby.
Reposition every 3-4 hr.
Offer explanations to parents.

ASSESSMENT—BIRTH TRAUMA

HEAD TRAUMA BIRTH INJURIES

Birth trauma	Assessment	Nursing interventions in the immediate neonatal period
Caput succedaneum	Soft, vaguely outlined swelling of scalp May cross sagittal suture lines	Explain to parents that swelling will subside in 2 or 3 days (see Client Infant Care Education: Caput Succedaneum and Cephalohematoma).
Cephalohematoma	Bleeding between cranial bone and its covering, the periosteum May appear bluish or bruised Does not cross limits of the bone	Explain to parents that swelling will subside in few weeks to 3 months. In the first few days place infant in side-lying position opposite from injury or in a prone position; area may be sensitive if touched for first few days.
Intracranial hemorrhage	Hemorrhage in various areas of brain caused by rupture of cerebral blood vessels	Assess for developing symptoms. Provide quiet environment, usually in isolette. Monitor temperature and respirations.

Continued

ASSESSMENT—BIRTH TRAUMA

HEAD TRAUMA BIRTH INJURIES—continued

Birth trauma	Assessment	Nursing interventions in the immediate neonatal period
	Low Apgar scores	
	Irregular respirations	
	Apneic episodes	
	Cold, pale, clammy skin	
	Lethargy	
	Signs of increasing intracranial pressure	
Facial paralysis	Mouth drawn to one side	Administer artificial tears as prescribed by physician.
	Eye on affected side may remain open	Provide small, frequent feedings, using soft nipple if sucking is difficult.
	Possibly unable to blink on affected side	
Arm paralysis (Erb's palsy)	Arm limp and internally rotated	Maintain proper position as prescribed.
	Grasp reflex present	Apply intermittent splinting as prescribed.
	Moro reflex lessened or absent on affected side	Perform daily passive range of motion exercises.
Fractures of clavicle, humerus, or femur	Decreased or absent mobility of affected arm or leg	Handle gently to minimize pain.
	Cries in pain when arm or leg moved	Immobilize by splinting.
	Local swelling	Maintain proper alignment.
		Arm on side of fractured clavicle may be held in place by pinning the sleeve to the shirt.

INTERVENTION

CLIENT INFANT-CARE EDUCATION: CAPUT SUCCEDANEUM AND CEPHALOHEMATOMA

Information

Caput Succedaneum
Swelling will disappear in several days. No special care is needed.

Cephalohematoma
Swelling may not disappear for days or weeks. Time is needed for absorption of the hematoma.

Position infant on the stomach or side opposite the hematoma. Infant may be irritable and fussy if he or she lies on the swollen area.

Be gentle when washing the area during the first several days.

Rationale

Parents may ask questions or show concern because of the head's swelling. The swelling occurs in the area that presented at the cervical os.

Cephalohematomas absorb spontaneously. Attempts to aspirate them may cause infection and thus are contraindicated.

If swelling is large, there may be pressure against the surrounding tissue, causing sensitivity.

NEONATAL SEPSIS

Newborns may be infected before they are born through the placenta or after the rupture of the membranes. Infection may also be acquired during passage through the birth canal and during exposure to the hospital environment.

ONGOING ASSESSMENT OF CLINICAL SIGNS OF SEPSIS IN THE NEWBORN

Subtle, nonspecific signs
"Is not doing well"
"Does not look right"
Nonspecific respiratory problems

Respiratory signs
Tachypnea
Apnea
Grunting

Gastrointestinal signs
Diarrhea
Abdominal distention
Vomiting
Poor sucking or feeding

Skin
Pallor, cyanosis, mottling
Rashes
Jaundice

Central nervous system
Temperature instability
Full or bulging fontanel
Irritability
Seizure activity

Fever is frequently absent

ASSESSMENT

COMMONLY OCCURRING PATHOGENS, TRANSMISSION, CHARACTERISTICS, AND NURSING CONSIDERATIONS IN NEONATAL SEPSIS

Pathogen	Transmission	Characteristics (assessment)	Nursing considerations
β-Hemolytic streptococci	In utero or after a long, difficult delivery (10% of mothers are vaginal carriers) Premature rupture of membranes Exposure to adult carrier	Early onset Low Apgar scores Respiratory distress Pneumonia at birth Sepsis Meningitis	Assist with septic workup. Assess for neurologic status: bulging fontanel, irritability, seizures, high-pitched cry. Measure head circumference. Administer antibiotic therapy as ordered.
Gonococcus	Contamination of infant's eyes with infected secretions from mother's vagina	On second or third day of life, serosanguineous discharge from eye, which becomes purulent (ophthalmia neonatorum) Ulceration and scarring of cornea, leading to blindness	Apply prophylactic medication to eyes at time of birth. Obtain smears for culture as ordered. Administer antibiotic as ordered.
Escherichia coli or other enteric pathogens	Gastrointestinal route through hands of caregiver Maternal fecal contamination at birth	(Serious problem in neonate requiring careful separation and isolation) Multiple loose stools Greenish or blood-tinged watery stools Weight loss Dehydration Sepsis Shock	Carefully isolate baby; when infection is confirmed, care for in a separate area with hand-washing and isolation facilities. Restrict exposure to new admissions. Administer antibiotics as ordered by the physician.

Chapter 18

HIGH-RISK NEONATAL CARE

Early identification of the infant at risk is often life-saving for the potentially compromised baby. Classification of a newborn as high risk may be the result of antepartal, intrapartal or neonatal risk factors. This chapter presents risk factors associated with premature and postmature infants.

CHARACTERISTICS OF PREMATURE INFANT

Periodic breathing with episodes of apnea
Thin, transparent skin
Abundant vernix
Fine, feathery hair
Little subcutaneous fat
Head large in relation to body
Limbs extended
Ear cartilages poorly developed
Clitoris prominent in female
Scrotum underdeveloped in male
Absent, weak, or ineffectual grasping, sucking, and swallowing
Unable to maintain body temperature

ASSESSMENT

IDENTIFICATION OF HIGH-RISK INFANT: ASSOCIATED FACTORS

ANTEPARTAL FACTORS

Maternal Characteristics

Age less than 15 or more than 35 yr

Low socioeconomic status

Unmarried

Family or marital conflicts

Emotional illness or family history of mental illness

Persistent ambivalence or conflicts about the pregnancy

Stature less than 5 feet

20% underweight or overweight

Malnutrition

Reproductive History

Parity greater than eight

Two or more previous abortions

Previous stillborn or neonatal death

Previous premature labor or low-birth-weight infant (<2500 g)

Previous excessively large infant (>4000 g)

Infant with isoimmunization or ABO incompatibility

Infant with congenital anomaly, genetic disorder, or birth damage

Preeclampsia or eclampsia

Uterine fibroids >5 cm or submucous

Abnormal Papanicolaou smear

Infertility

Prior cesarean section

Prior fetal malpresentations

Contracted pelvis

Ovarian masses

Genital tract abnormalities (incompetent cervix, subseptate or bicornate uterus)

Pregnancy occurring 3 mon or less after last delivery

Previous prolonged labor or significant dystocia

Substance Abuse

Drugs

Alcohol

Heavy smoking (>2 packs/day)

Medical Problems

Chronic hypertension

Renal disease (pyelonephritis, glomerulonephritis, polycystic kidney)

Diabetes mellitus (classes B to F)

Heart disease (aortic insufficiency, pulmonary hypertension, diastolic murmur, cardiac enlargement, heart failure, dysrhythmia)

Sickle cell trait or disease

Anemias with hemoglobin <9 g and hematocrit <32%

Continued

ASSESSMENT

IDENTIFICATION OF HIGH-RISK INFANT: ASSOCIATED FACTORS—continued

ANTEPARTAL FACTORS—cont'd

Pulmonary disease (tuberculosis, chronic obstructive pulmonary disease)

Endocrine disorders (hypothyroidism or hyperthyroidism, family history of cretinism, adrenal or pituitary problems)

Gastrointestinal or liver disease

Epilepsy

Malignancy (including leukemia and Hodgkin's disease)

Complications of Present Pregnancy

Low or excessive weight gain

Hypertension (mean arterial pressure >90, blood pressure 140/90, increase >30 mm Hg systolic or >20 mm Hg diastolic)

Recurrent glycosuria and abnormal fasting blood sugar or glucose tolerance test

Uterine size inappropriate for gestational age (either too large or too small)

Recurrent urinary tract infections

Severe varicosities or thrombophlebitis

Recurrent vaginal bleeding

Premature rupture of membranes

Multiple pregnancy

Hydramnios with a single fetus

Rh negative with a rising titer

Late or no prenatal care

Exposure to teratogens (medications, x-ray, radioactive isotopes)

Viral infections (rubella, cytomegalovirus, herpes, mumps, rubeola, chickenpox, shingles, smallpox, vaccinia, influenza, poliomyelitis, hepatitis, Western equine encephalitis, coxsackie virus B)

Syphilis, especially late pregnancy

Bacterial infections (gonorrhea, tuberculosis, listeriosis, severe acute infection)

Protozoan infections (toxoplasmosis, malaria)

Postmaturity

Anemia with hemoglobin of 9 g or less

Severe preeclampsia, eclampsia

Abnormal contraction stress test

Falling urinary estriol levels

INTRAPARTUM FACTORS

Complications of Labor and Delivery

Labor longer than 24 hr in primigravida

Labor longer than 12 hr in multigravida

Second stage longer than 1 hr

Ruptured membranes more than 24 hr

Abnormal presentation or position

Heavy sedation or injudicious anesthesia

Maternal fever or infection

Placenta previa or abruptio placentae

Cesarean section

Meconium-stained amniotic fluid

Fetal distress caused by monitoring or scalp blood sampling

Prolapsed cord

High forceps or midforceps delivery, difficult or operative delivery

Premature labor

Severe preeclampsia, eclampsia

Precipitous labor less than 3 hr

Elective induction

Oxytocin (Pitocin) augmentation

Immediate Problems of Infant

Malformation or other significant abnormality

Birth injury

Asphyxia (Apgar <6 at 5 min)

NEONATAL FACTORS

Characteristics of Infant

Preterm or premature

SGA or LGA

Birth weight <5½ pounds or >9 pounds

Low-set ears

Enlargement of one or both kidneys

Single palmar crease

Single umbilical artery

Small head size

Clinical Problems

Feeding problems

Anemia

Hyperbilirubinemia

Temperature instability

Respiratory distress

Hypoglycemia

Polycythemia

Sepsis

Rh or ABO incompatibilities

Hypocalcemia

Persistent cyanosis

Shock

Seizures

Heart murmur

INTERVENTION

COMPARISON OF NURSING INTERVENTIONS FOR INFANTS OF VARYING GESTATIONAL AGE GROUPS

Classification	Assessment of clinical signs	Potential problems	Nursing interventions
Small for gestational age (intrauterine growth retardation [IUGR])	Loose, dry skin Vernix often decreased or absent Decrease in subcutaneous tissue and fat Sunken abdomen Thin, yellow, dull umbilical cord Sparse scalp hair Wide-eyed look	Increased risk of morbidity and mortality Related to abnormalities of fetus or pregnancy Prone to asphyxia at birth Prone to meconium aspiration Temperature instability Polycythemia Hypothermia Hypoglycemia	Nurses and doctors skilled in resuscitation present at birth Blood glucose evaluation on admission and every 2-4 hr Provision of caloric and fluid requirements Early feeding if hypoglycemic Provision of thermal environment
Large for gestational age	If infant of diabetic mother (IDM): Fat and enlarged appearance Ruddiness	Often the infant of a diabetic mother Other factors: heredity; males are larger than females; occurs in second or third pregnancies	Assessment of gestational age in relation to birth weight Assessment for complications

	Puffy appearance Early lethargy Irritability, jitteriness, tremors	Prone to birth injuries, cephalohematoma, ecchymosis Hypoglycemia Hyperbilirubinemia Polycythemia If IDM: congenital anomalies	Monitoring of temperature and respiratory status Frequent glucose assessment Provision of glucose, fluid, and caloric intake based on condition of infant
Postmature	May have symptoms of IUGR (see above) or of infant 1 to 3 wk old Lanugo absent Abundant scalp hair Long fingernails Cracked parchment or desquamating skin Long, thin appearance Worried look	Prone to uterine hypoxia related to decreasing efficiency of the placenta Meconium aspiration Hypoglycemia Polycythemia	Nurses and doctors skilled in resuscitation present at birth Blood glucose evaluation on admission

NURSING CARE PLAN

HIGH-RISK INFANT

Goals (expected outcomes)	Interventions	Rationale	Evaluation
INEFFECTIVE THERMOREGULATION—RELATED TO IMMATURE TEMPERATURE CONTROL, INFECTION, DECREASED SUBCUTANEOUS TISSUE			
Infant's temperature will remain within normal limits (97.7° to 98.6° F axillary).	Place infant in isolette or radiant warmer or wrap well in an open crib. Avoid chilling infant when removed from warming unit.	Preterm infant has high skin surface relative to body mass, which promotes heat loss, and has a small subcutaneous fat layer. Promotes a neutral thermal environment in which the infant's core temperature is normal and oxygen use and calorie output is minimal.	Temperature is within normal parameters (97.7° to 98.6° F axillary). Mechanical temperature of isolette or radiant warmer is within set parameters.
ALTERED NUTRITION: LESS THAN BODY REQUIREMENTS—RELATED TO INABILITY TO INGEST ADEQUATE NUTRIENTS BECAUSE OF IMMATURE SUCKING ABILITY, WEAKNESS, OR FATIGUE			
Infant will ingest adequate formula or breast milk (specify amount).	Maintain intravenous lines. Offer enteral feedings when infant is stable as evidenced by:	Oral feedings are contraindicated if tachypnea is present because of danger of aspiration.	Infant tolerates formula without vomiting, distention of abdomen, or

		changes in heart rate or blood pressure.
Infant will demonstrate steady weight gain (6-8 ounces/wk).	Temperature neutral	
	Normal breathing	
	Good color and cry	
	Offer amounts determined by infant's size, age, condition.	
	Feed for 20-30 min only to avoid tiring infant.	
	Gavage feed infants more than 32 wk old or more than 1650 g with poor sucking.	
	Conserve neonate's energy.	
	Amount and method of feeding are ordered by the physician according to size and condition of the infant.	
	Coordination of sucking and swallowing occurs at approximately 32 to 34 wk gestation.	Infant begins to make attempts at sucking and swallowing during gavage.
	Intermittent gavage feeding through the mouth is a safe means of feeding for infants who are too weak to suck effectively or who become excessively tired, listless, or cyanotic during feedings.	Infant has steady weight gain.

Continued

Nursing Care Plan

HIGH-RISK INFANT—continued

Goals (expected outcomes)	Interventions	Rationale	Evaluation
IMPAIRMENT IN SKIN INTEGRITY—RELATED TO IMMATURE SKIN STRUCTURE AND USE OF TAPE TO FASTEN MONITORING DEVICES AND INTRAVENOUS LINES			
Infant's skin remains intact without evidence of irritation or trauma.	Cleanse skin with water. Use transpore tape to secure items to skin.	Skin of the preterm infant is thin, sensitive, and fragile and is easily damaged.	Infant's skin remains intact.
	Apply protective covering to skin before taping. Exert great care when handling skin. Place on water pillow or fleece. Change position every 2-3 hr.	Damaged skin provides an entrance for pathogens and resultant infections.	
ALTERED PARENTING—RELATED TO INTERRUPTION OF BONDING PROCESS OR LACK OF PARENTAL KNOWLEDGE			
Parents express feelings and concerns about the infant and his or her progress.	Give parents adequate preparation and information when visiting infant.	There is evidence that the physical and emotional separation of the parent(s) and infant inter-	Parents share their concerns and anxieties about their infant. Parents visit at times when

		they can become involved in infant's care.
Parents visit infant as frequently as possible.	Answer parents' questions and allow expressions of concern. Provide photographs and emphasize specialness of newborn.	Parents call their infant by name and verbalize interest in infant as an individual.
Parents demonstrate care for infant as appropriate.	Demonstrate care of newborn when parents show readiness.	Parental involvement, assisted by the nurse, helps parents to cope with care of their infant and to assume care when infant is discharged.

INEFFECTIVE BREATHING PATTERN—RELATED TO IMMATURE BREATHING CENTER, IMPAIRED GAS EXCHANGE, DECREASED LUNG EXPANSION OR FATIGUE

Infant's breathing is unlabored, and periods of apnea are within normal limits (state parameters). Infant's breathing rate is within normal limits (state parameters).	Observe, record, and report signs and symptoms of respiratory distress: Tachypnea Cyanosis Retractions Grunting Nasal flaring Diminished breath sounds	Without surfactant the preterm infant has difficulty keeping the lungs inflated. Atelectasis and hypoxemia may result. The preterm baby also has weak chest wall muscles.	Respirations are regular and the rate within normal limits.

Continued

NURSING CARE PLAN

HIGH-RISK INFANT—continued

Goals (expected outcomes)	Interventions	Rationale	Evaluation
INEFFECTIVE BREATHING PATTERN—RELATED TO IMMATURE BREATHING CENTER, IMPAIRED GAS EXCHANGE, DECREASED LUNG EXPANSION OR FATIGUE—cont'd			
	Keep airway open by suctioning and positioning. Administer O_2 along with appropriate monitoring of blood gas values. Change position frequently. Gently stimulate to breathe during periods of apnea. Monitor heart and respiratory rates and number and length of apneic periods.	O_2 therapy provides adequate O_2 to the tissues.	
FLUID VOLUME DEFICIT—RELATED TO INSENSIBLE WATER LOSS, INADEQUATE FLUID INTAKE, OR INFECTIOUS PROCESS			
Infant exhibits no symptoms of dehydration. Infant loses minimum birth weight.	Maintain intravenous lines and monitor closely for infiltration.	Providing adequate fluids is very important for the preterm infant because	Intravenous site is free of infiltration signs. Intravenous fluids are flow-

Administer correct fluid and correct amount per hour. Record total intake per shift and daily. Observe for signs of dehydration: Skin turgor Urinary output Condition of fontanel Temperature Weight loss Mucous membrane Urinary specific gravity	...ing at correct rates as ordered by physician. his or her extracellular water content is higher than that of a fullterm infant. The preterm infant's kidneys are underdeveloped and are very vulnerable to water loss.	Minimal weight loss. No symptoms of dehydration.

DRUG GUIDES

BROMOCRIPTINE MESYLATE (PARLODEL)

Ergot derivative; stimulates dopamine receptors; commonly used in treatment of Parkinson's disease

Obstetric action: Inhibits prolactin secretion, postpartum physiolgoic lactation, and breast engorgement

Postpartum administration
>   Average dosage: 2.5 mg b.i.d. for 14 to 21 days
>   *Special note:*
>>   It must *not* be administered until vital signs are stable. Therapy must begin a minimum of 4 hr after delivery. Administer orally with food.

Maternal contraindications: Uncontrolled hypertension, pregnancy-induced hypertension, allergy to ergot alkaloids

Potential side effects and complications: Symptomatic transient hypotension, dizziness, nausea, severe headaches, blurred vision, seizures, stroke, hypertension during second week of therapy

Nursing implications
- Assess client's medical and prenatal history to identify contraindications to administration.
- Monitor status closely after administering initial dose (most common time of negative reaction to drug is 10 to 20 min after first dose).
- Assess client's blood pressure and general status before each administration and/or every 4 hr while awake.
- Hold medication and notify physician if client becomes hypotensive or hypertensive or complains of other above-listed signs or symptoms of side effects.
- Ambulate client with assistance if necessary.

Client teaching
- Advise client to continue taking drug, as ordered, with meals or milk; avoid alcohol.
- Advise her to store drug in tightly closed container.
- Stress importance of return visit to physician as instructed.
- Discuss possibility of pregnancy's occurring before reinitiation of menses.
- Recommend use of barrier contraceptives during postpartum period; use of oral contraceptives is contraindicated.

- Inform about possible transient mild-to-moderate rebound engorgement when discontinuing drug.
- Emphasize need to notify physician promptly if she experiences one or more episodes of severe headaches, blurred vision, dizziness, nausea, chest pain.

BUTORPHANOL TARTRATE (STADOL)

A synthetic nonnarcotic analgesic for relief of moderate to severe pain.

Obstetric action: Effective for pain relief in labor, although the exact mechanism of the drug is unknown. It is thought to act on the subcortical portion of the central nervous system.

Labor and delivery administration: Average dose is 2 mg IM every 3-4 hr or 1 mg IV every 3-4 hr.

Maternal contraindications: History of hypersensitivity; should be used with caution in woman delivering a premature baby.

Potential side effects and complications: The most frequent reactions are nausea, clamminess, and sweating. Less frequent reactions are headaches, vertigo, a floating feeling, dizziness, lethargy, confusion, and light-headedness.

Nursing implications
- Assess client's history and initial data base for hypersensitivity to butorphanol.
- If analgesic is given IV, administer it slowly just as a contraction is subsiding to minimize effect of rapid absorption on fetus.
- If giving intramuscularly, administer deeply into muscle (given IM if there is no IV line).
- Instruct client to remain in bed with side rails up; have signal cord within reach.
- Observe for maternal side effects (decreased respirations, increased blood pressure, nausea, increased perspiration).
- Evaluate effectiveness of pain relief.
- Assess client's bladder at least every 2 hr for distention and encourage her to void.
- Assess fetal monitor strip for reactivity and variability.
- Assess newborn respiratory status and muscle tone at delivery.

EPIDURAL MORPHINE SULFATE

An exogenous opiate that weakens signals to the brain by binding opiate receptors at many sites in the central nervous system, the brain (cortex), brain stem (thalamus), and spinal cord (dorsal horn), altering both the perception and emotional response to pain through an unknown mechanism.

Obstetric action: Intense analgesic effect from direct action on the opiate receptors of the spinal cord rather than from systematic absorption. Onset is slower, but duration of analgesia is longer.

Dosage: 5-7.5 mg—provides analgesia for approximately 24 hours.

Maternal contraindications: Allergy to morphine.

Potential side effects and complications:
Pruritus
Itching may be mild or severe; generally begins within 3 hours and lasts up to 10 hours. Naloxone (0.1 to 0.2 mg IV bolus or infusion of 0.4 to 0.6 mg/hr) will relieve symptoms; if client can tolerate itching, she can avoid taking naloxone, which counteracts the pain relief benefit.
Nausea or vomiting
Can occur 4 to 7 hours after morphine injection. Naloxone alleviates the symptoms without affecting the analgesic effect of the epidural morphine. Diphenhydramine (Benadryl) or trimethobenzamide (Tigan) can be given.
Urinary retention
Onset is early and lasts 14 to 16 hours; not usually a problem since client has Foley catheter in place.
Respiratory depression
Rare, with rate <12%. Can occur during first 1 to 2 hours or as late as 8 to 16 hours after instillation; less likely to occur if mother is in semi-Fowler's position.
Newborn effects
Since the morphine is injected into the catheter after the infant is born, there are no adverse effects.

Nursing implications:
• Assess for client's sensitivity to narcotics on admission.
• Have a vial of naloxone (Narcan) (1 ml, 0.4 mg) readily available for immediate administration in case of respiratory depression.

- Answer questions about analgesia and anticipate questions when possible.
- Assess respiratory function hourly for 24 hours, as well as client's level of consciousness or sedation and color of mucous membranes; may use apnea monitor for 24 hours to determine if there is a decrease in respirations.
- Assess pain relief and notify anesthesiologist if not adequate.
- Observe for allergic reactions such as itching, edema, or respiratory difficulties.
- Observe for nausea or vomiting.
- Administer comfort measures such as lotions, cool or warm packs, cool or light clothing, or diversional activities.
- Administer medications such as diphenhydramine or naloxone as ordered to alleviate side effects.
- Monitor output if Foley catheter in place; ensure it is patent and draining (assist client with bedpan or to bathroom when Foley catheter is discontinued and motor and sensory function have returned).
- Instruct the client to rest (since tendency is to be active much sooner after cesarean delivery).

ERGONOVINE MALEATE (ERGOTRATE)

Principal oxytocic alkaloid of ergot, a fungus that grows on rye and other grains.

Obstetric action: Induces uterine muscle contractions and exerts an effect that lasts for hours. After its administration, contraction of uterine muscle occurs rapidly and is sustained; valuable aid in control of postpartum bleeding.

Postpartum administration: May be administered orally or parenterally. It is available in tablet form in doses of 0.2 mg to be given orally and in 1 ml ampules containing 0.2 mg (1/320 gr) for intramuscular (IM) or IV administration. Usual dose is 0.2 mg (1/320 gr).

Maternal contraindications: Generally contraindicated in women who have hypertension, particularly PIH.

Potential side effects and complications: Dizziness, headache, tinnitus, dysrhythmias, chest pain, palpitations, hypertension (if given IV), dyspnea.

Nursing implications:
- Assess client's medical and prenatal history to identify contraindications to administration.
- Monitor uterine fundal height and consistency; monitor lochia for bleeding, amount, character, and odor.
- Assess blood pressure before and after drug administration and every 15 min if client is hypotensive or hypertensive.
- Observe for adverse effects or symptoms of ergot toxicity: nausea, vomiting, diarrhea, changes in blood pressure, chest pain, numb and cold extremities, dyspnea, weak pulse, excitability to convulsions, delirium, hallucinations.
- Instruct client that uterine cramping is expected and that an analgesia order can be obtained from the physician if needed.

ERYTHROMYCIN (ILOTYCIN) OPHTHALMIC OINTMENT

Provides bacterocidal or bacterostatic protection, depending on the organisms and the concentration of the drug.

Neonatal action: A single dose (about ½ inch [2 cm] long strand of ointment) is placed along the lower conjunctival sac of each eye (from inner canthus outward). It is preferable that the newborn have some time to attach with the family before the ointment is instilled.

Neonatal contraindications: Contraindicated if there is known history of hypersensitivity.

Potential side effects and complications: Chemical conjunctivitis occurs in approximately 20% of neonates; may interfere with ability to focus and may cause edema and inflammation. Side effects usually disappear within 24 to 48 hours.

Nursing implications:
- Wash hands before instilling eye ointment.
- Wear gloves if initial bath has not been given.
- Gently open eyelids to prevent undue trauma.
- Do not irrigate eyes after instillation.
- Observe for hypersensitivity.

HEPARIN SODIUM INJECTION

Sterile solution derived from porcine intestinal mucosa, standardized for use as anticoagulant.

Obstetric action: Inhibits reactions that lead to clotting of blood and formation of fibrin clots; acts at multiple sites in the normal coagulation systems; prolongs clotting time; has no effect on existing clots but prevents extension of old clots and formation of new ones.

Postpartum administration: IV or subcutaneous (SC), 5000 to 30,000 U; may be ordered as a drip over 24 hr. Prophylactic dose: 5000 U SC every 12 hr.

Maternal contraindications: Sensitivity to heparin.

Potential side effects and complications: Hemorrhage (chief complication); hypersensitivity reactions with chills, fever and urticaria; possible local irritation, mild pain, and hematoma formation with intramuscular injection; acute thrombocytopenia purpura, alopecia; long-term use during pregnancy associated with maternal osteopenia, possibly from low vitamin D.

Nursing implications:
- Do not administer heparin intramuscularly.
- Order laboratory tests (coagulation time) as ordered by primary health care provider (usually every 4 hr).
- Report results of coagulation tests of prothrombin activity before start of therapy.
- Monitor closely for hemorrhage.
- Rotate administration site.
- Do not massage administration site.
- Mother may continue to breast-feed.

MAGNESIUM SULFATE (50%)

Primary action is to compete with calcium to block the reuptake of acetylcholine at the synapses. Its anticonvulsant mechanism of action is still not understood and is controversial.

Obstetric action: To control seizure activity.

Preparation and administration:
Intravenous route
1. Prepare *loading dose:* 4 g magnesium sulfate added to 240 ml D_5W. Administer by piggyback method (using an infusion pump or controller) over a 15- to 20-min period.
2. Maintenance of a therapeutic level requires an intravenous

(IV) infusion of 3 g/hr. (Effects of drug last 30 min if given intravenously and 3-4 hr if given intramuscularly).

Combination of intramuscular (IM) and intravenous (IV) routes
1. Administer the *loading dose* of 4 g magnesium sulfate IV over 20 min and simultaneously administer 10 mg magnesium sulfate IM (5 g deeply into each buttock). If drug is injected into subcutaneous tissue, necrosis will occur.
2. Give 5 g of magnesium sulfate every 4 hr (deep IM). The IV dose is given to obtain therapeutic levels rapidly (4-7 mg/dl).

Maternal contraindications: Magnesium sulfate should be withheld if the patellar reflex disappears, respirations are <12-14 per minute, or if urinary output is <30 ml/hr.

Potential side effects and complications: Early signs of magnesium intoxication include the following:

Hot all over   Depression of reflexes
Flushing   Hypotension
Thirst   Muscle flaccidity
Sweating

Later signs of hypermagnesemia are as follows:
Central nervous system depression (respirations <12, decreased reflexes)
Respiratory paralysis (magnesium, 10-12 mg/dl)
Circulatory collapse (dose >15 mg/dl)
Note: If the above occur, calcium gluconate is the antidote.

Nursing implications:
- Assess deep tendon reflexes hourly (if client receiving continuous infusion).
- Monitor client's blood pressure, pulse, and respiration every 15-30 min; report if respirations <12-14 or hypotension occurs.
- Monitor intake and output every hour; if output is <30 ml/hr, notify physician and anticipate decreasing or discontinuing the magnesium sulfate.
- Continuously monitor client's orientation to person, place, and time.
- Assess client for complaints of headache, nausea, vomiting, or epigastric pain.
- Monitor fetus intermittently or continuously as indicated by physician's order.

- Continue seizure precautions (e.g., padded side rail, quiet environment).
- Keep the antidote, calcium gluconate (10% solution), at client's bedside.

MEPERIDINE HYDROCHLORIDE (DEMEROL)

A narcotic analgesic that interferes with pain impulses at the subcortical level of the brain; used during labor for analgesic effect.

Obstetric action: Enhances analgesia by altering the physiologic response to pain; suppresses anxiety and apprehension of labor.

Labor and delivery administration: Average dose is 50-100 mg intramuscularly (IM) every 3-4 hr or 25-50 mg by slow intravenous (IV) push every 3-4 hr.

Maternal contraindications: Hypersensitivity to meperidine, asthma, central nervous system or respiratory depression, nonreassuring fetal heart rate patterns.

Potential side effects and complications: Respiratory depression, nausea and vomiting, dry mouth, drowsiness, dizziness, flushing, transient hypotension, bradycardia, palpitation.

Nursing implications:
- Assess client's history, initial data base for history of hypersensitivity.
- If given IV, administer meperidine slowly just as contraction subsides to minimize effect of rapid absorption on fetus.
- If given IM, administer deeply into muscle (given IM if there is no IV line).
- Instruct client to remain in bed with bed rails up; have signal cord within her reach.
- Observe client for maternal side effects such as dizziness or nausea.
- Evaluate effectiveness of drug in relieving pain of labor.
- Assess client's bladder for distention (at least every 2 hr) and encourage her to void.
- Assess fetal monitor strip for reactivity and variability.
- Assess newborn respiratory status and muscle tone at delivery.

METHYLERGONOVINE MALEATE (METHERGINE)

Ergot alkaloid that stimulates contraction of smooth muscle.

Obstetric action: Stimulates uterus to contract, thus clamping uterine blood vessels to prevent hemorrhage; also has vasconstrictive effect on all blood vessels (especially larger arteries), causing elevation of blood pressure.

Postpartum administration:: Usual dose is 0.2 mg (PO) after delivery and every 4 hr times six doses; dose may be repeated every 2-4 hr if necessary.
Special note: This drug usually is not given IV if client has elevated blood pressure. If it is administered to a hypertensive woman, her blood pressure must be monitored continuously.

Maternal contraindications: Pregnancy, induction of labor, hepatic or renal disease, threatened spontaneous abortion, uterine sepsis, cardiac disease, hypertension, and obliterative vascular disease.

Potential side effects and complications: Hypertension (particularly if given IV), nausea, vomiting, headache, bradycardia, dizziness, tinnitus, abdominal cramps, palpitations, dyspnea, chest pain, and allergic reactions.

Nursing implications:
- Assess client's medical and prenatal history to identify contrain-dications to administration.
- Monitor uterine fundus for height, consistency, and lochial amount, character, and odor.
- Assess blood pressure before administration.
- Assess blood pressure after administration and every 15 min if client is hypotensive or hypertensive.
- Observe for adverse effects or symptoms of ergot toxicity (nausea, vomiting, diarrhea, changes in blood pressure, chest pain, numb and cold extremities, dyspnea, weak pulse, excitability, convul-sions, delirium, hallucinations).
- Instruct client that uterine cramping is expected and that an analgesia order can be obtained from the physician if needed.

NALOXONE HYDROCHLORIDE (NARCAN)

A narcotic antagonist that reverses respiratory depression in-duced by a variety of narcotics.

Obstetric action: Used in clients who have received epidural (intraspinal) morphine to decrease or relieve completely its side effects.

Postpartum (after epidural morphine) administration: Average dose is 0.1-0.2 mg IV repeated as necessary if respiratory depression is noted.

Maternal contraindications: Known client hypersensitivity to the drug; use cautiously if client is suspected of being physically dependent on opioids.

Potential side effects and complications: Hypotension, hypertension, ventricular tachycardia, fibrillation, and pulmonary edema have been reported most often in clients with preexisting cardiovascular disorders or who have received other drugs that may have similar adverse cardiovascular effects. Abrupt reversal of narcotic depression may result in nausea, vomiting, sweating, tachycardia, increased blood pressure, and tremulousness. In postoperative clients, larger than usual doses of naloxone may result in significant reversal of analgesia and in excitement. Seizures have been reported infrequently.

Nursing implications:
- A vial of naloxone (1 ml, 0.4 mg) must be readily available at the nurse's station for immediate administration if respiratory depression occurs.
- An airway, oxygen suction, and emergency life support drugs should be available.
- Nurses caring for these clients should be currently certified in community cardiopulmonary resuscitation (CPR) or basic life support (BLS).
- Since naloxone may be present in breast milk, the client should not breast-feed until the epidural analgesia has ended.
- Naloxone should not be mixed with any other drug unless its effects on the chemical and physical stability of the solution have been established.

OXYTOCIN (PITOCIN)

Synthetic hormone that stimulates rhythmic contractions of the uterine muscle. The onset of action is immediate. When properly administered, oxytocin should stimulate contractions comparable to those seen in normal spontaneous labor.

Obstetric action: Exerts a selective stimulatory effect on the smooth muscle of the uterus and of the blood vessels. It affects the myometrial cells by increasing the excitability of the muscle cell, which increases the strength of the muscle contraction and supports propagation of the contraction, i.e., movement of the contraction from one myometrial cell to the next.

Uterine sensitivity to oxytocin increases gradually as gestation continues toward term and increases sharply before parturition. Oxytocin is used for the initiation or improvement of uterine contractions for clients with medical indications, when birth is in the best interest of both mother and fetus, for uterine inertia, for afterbirth of the placenta, to control postpartum hemorrhage, and in inevitable or incomplete abortion.

Administration for induction or augmentation of labor: Average dosage is usually 10 U (1 ml) Pitocin added to 1000 ml of IV electrolyte solution delivered to the mainline through a secondary line.

Maternal contraindications: Hypersensitivity, significant cephalopelvic disproportion, prolonged use in uterine inertia or severe toxemia, abnormal fetal presentation or position, where surgical interventions are favored for the maternal client and fetus, elective induction, prior classic cesarean section; active genital herpes, rigid unripe cervix, presence of fetal stress and/or distress.

Potential side effects and complications: Hyperstimulation of the uterus results in hypercontractibility, which in turn may cause (1) abruptio placentae; (2) decreased uterine blood flow, which can cause fetal hypoxia; (3) rapid labor and delivery, which can result in lacerations of cervix, vagina, and perineum and uterine atony, fetal trauma; (4) uterine rupture; or (5) water intoxication, i.e., nausea, vomiting, hypotension, tachycardia, or cardiac arrhythmia, if oxytocin is given in electrolyte-free solution.

Nursing implications:
- Assess client's medical, prenatal, labor history, and fetal monitor to identify reasons for administration and potential contraindications.
- Prepare and begin infusion as ordered by physician.

- Monitor uterine activity before increasing oxytocin infusion for frequency, duration, intensity, and shape of contractions and resting tone of uterus.
- Assess FHR for tachycardia, bradycardia, late and severe variable decelerations.

Note: If there is excessive uterine activity (contractions closer than 2 minutes and lasting longer than 90 seconds) or a non-reassuring fetal heart tracing, turn the Pitocin infusion OFF, begin intrauterine resuscitation, and notify the physician immediately (see Nursing Procedure: Intrauterine Resuscitation.

- Monitor maternal blood pressure and pulse each time before increasing oxytocin infusion drip rate.
- Document all maternal and fetal observations on the monitor tracing and in the nurses' notes.
- Monitor and document intake and output.
- Be alert for signs of uterine rupture which occurs infrequently, including excruciating pain, cessation of contractions, vaginal hemorrhage (may occur), signs of hypovolemic shock, and loss of FHR.

Note: Oxytocin has an antidiuretic effect; therefore, large volumes of nonelectrolyte solutions are avoided. This eliminates the risk of water intoxication.

PHYTONADIONE (AQUAMEPHYTON)

Aqueous colloidal solution of vitamin K. Possesses the same type and degree of activity as naturally occurring vitamin K. Necessary for blood clotting.

Neonatal action: Used as prophylaxis and treatment of hemorrhagic disease of the newborn. Promotes liver formation of several clotting factors. At birth, the newborn does not have the bacteria in the colon necessary for synthesizing fat-soluble vitamin K, so prothrombin levels are decreased for 5 to 8 days of life.

Neonatal administration: A one-time prophylactic dosage of 0.5 to 1.0 mg is administered intramuscularly into the anterior or lateral thigh. May be given after delivery as a part of the initial care or a little later during the assessment process done by the mother-infant nurse or nursery nurse. May need repeat dose in 6 to 8 hours if mother was on anticoagulants.

Neonatal contraindications: Hypersensitivity to any component of this medication.

Potential side effects and contraindications: Pain and edema may occur at the site of injection. There may be allergic reaction (rash and urticaria). Some newborns may develop hyperbilirubinemia and jaundice if a larger dose is given.

Nursing implications:
- Store in a dark place to protect vitamin K from light before use. The drug is photosensitive and decomposes with loss of potency on exposure to light.
- Wash hands prior to administering.
- Wear gloves if initial newborn bath not yet given.
- Observe for signs of local inflammation.
- Assess for bleeding, which may occur as generalized ecchymoses or as bleeding from cord, nose, or gastrointestinal tract.
- Assess for jaundice.

RH_o (D) IMMUNE GLOBULIN (HUMAN) (RHOGAM)

A sterile concentrated solution of specific immunoglobulin (IgG) containing anti-Rh_o (D) prepared from human fractionated plasma.

Obstetric action: Immune globulin acts by suppressing the specific immune response of unsensitized Rh-negative mothers to Rh-positive red blood cells (RBCs). It prevents hemolytic disease in their Rh-positive newborns.

Administration: Rh_o (D) immunoglobulin is administered intramuscularly.
1. One vial (300 μg) is given for antepartum prophylaxis (at approximately 28 wk).
2. One vial (50 μg) is given after amniocentesis, miscarriage, abortion, or etopic pregnancy or beyond 13 weeks of gestation. If pregnancy terminates before 13 weeks, a vial of MICRhoGAM may be used.
3. One vial is given for postpartum prophylaxis within 72 hr of delivery if tests indicate no sensitization has occurred.

Potential side effects and complications: Reactions are infrequent and mild and are confined to the area of injection. Systemic reactions are rare.

Nursing implications:
- The nurse is responsible for checking the blood types and Rh status of every pregnant client.
- The nurse will have a standing order or will obtain an order from the primary physician to do all of the following unless the father is known to be Rh negative.
  - Give one dose of prophylactic Rh immunoglobulin (RhIG) (300 μg) to every unsensitized Rh-negative client at 28 weeks gestation unless the father of the fetus is known to be Rh negative.
  - Do an Rh blood workup on both mother and infant at the time of the delivery to determine the blood type and Rh of the neonate, and give one prophylactic dose of RhIG as soon as possible after delivery to affected mothers.
  - Give every Rh-negative unsensitized woman who aborts at least 50 μg of RhIG.
  - Administer RhIG (300 μg) to every Rh-negative, unimmunized woman undergoing amniocentesis.
- The nurse will be asked to order a Betke-Kleihauer stain to assess the amount of fetal blood in the maternal circulation; this result will assist the physician in adjusting the dosage of Rh_o (D) immune globulin.

INDEX